Tom Patire, creator of CDT® and Training for Life™ and author of *Tom Patire's Personal Protection Handbook,* has trained thousands of law enforcement officials, security professionals, and ordinary men, women, and children. Here are some comments from satisfied clients.

"Tom Patire is the finest and most sought-after instructor I have ever had the privilege to learn from. I cannot recommend a finer person or a more qualified instructor to your organization."

—Robert J. Hammond, deputy U.S. marshal

"I never imagined that someone of my size and strength would be able to disarm and control a very large, enraged individual. These simple and very effective techniques were easy to learn and use. I strongly recommend and encourage everyone to take Tom Patire's personal protection program. It left me confident and sure of how to live a safer life, whether it be at work or at home."

—Jose Petitclerc, flight attendant

"I am a mother to two children, ages 7 and 15. What goes on in the newspapers, the news, high schools, and around the corner at your local convenience store is shocking, but I believe in this course. It has given me the knowledge to defend against anyone safely, safely for both parties."

—Mrs. Nico Gagne, mother

"CDT Family Protection is the first program to address the family as a unit. What's that worth? It's priceless! I would like to congratulate Tom Patire and praise him for developing a system for the everyday person. Most self-protection systems take years of training, but his expertise and ingenuity paved the way for the ultimate training courses for the masses—Training for Life."

—Mike Swain, four-time Olympian and world judo champion

"As a trained martial artist I always knew I could protect myself but was always worried as to how to protect my family. Your Training for Life concept answered all my questions and fears. I just wanted to say thanks."

—Kerry Roy, martial arts instructor

"Your realistic look and techniques on child safety sold me on your program. Taking your program has allowed me to go from being just a mother and a provider to a safety-conscious protector."

—Beth Newton, mother

"Tom Patire's Training for Life taught me protection is more than being tough—it's about being smart!"

—Lee Ellen Ward, grandmother

"I have had the pleasure of attending Tom's enlightening seminars on living a safer life. I find him articulate, intelligent, and highly skilled. His Training for Life course is a must for anybody and everybody!"

—Dr. Timothy Geary, assistant superintendent of schools

"Although you were highly recommended to me by other state and federal agencies, I was not prepared for the professionalism, experience, and instructor qualification that I personally witnessed during my attendance at your program. Tom Patire is in a class of his own!"

—Alan J. Robinson, security executive

"Tom Patire is one of the most professional and highly skilled people I have ever had the privilege to train under."

—James Monaghan Jr., police lieutenant

"Tom Patire's Training for Life was the perfect safety program for all my employees. It was entertaining, educational, and timely and has created an aura of safety in our workplace."

—James Miller, security director

"I would like to thank you for the outstanding instruction that you have provided for our agency. Your dedication to assisting law enforcement agencies continues to benefit all the agents in the field."

—Thomas Modafferi, U.S. postal inspector

"Tom Patire's program left me confident in my training. I believe anyone from a college student to a grandparent can greatly benefit from his system."

—Diana Tipton, mother

"I am very grateful to you and your system. It helped me rescue my teenage daughter, who was being victimized by an older man. Before attending your class I did not know what to do. Afterward I was confident in your beliefs and training. End result: I saved my daughter!"

—Donna Koshad, mother

"I enrolled in Tom Patire's program to get some safety tips but left energized and vitalized under the Training for Life philosophy. This program is a must for women of all ages."

—Karen Colon, mother

"Tom Patire's program has given me more confidence in my ability to protect myself and to be more conscious about my surroundings. I am small in stature, but Training for Life made me feel like I was ten feet tall."

—Mary Case, clerk

"I'm 46 years old, I have a progressive and disabling disease, and I'm doing just fine! I understand better than many people what it is to live with uncertainty. It is why Tom Patire's programs *are* empowering and important for everyone. For me, it boils down to Tom's well-chosen words: I'm 'Training for Life.' "

—Pat Feahr

TOM PATIRE'S

PERSONAL
PROTECTION

HANDBOOK

Absolutely Everything
You Need to Know
to Keep Yourself, Your Family,
and Your Assets Safe

TOM PATIRE

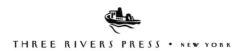

THREE RIVERS PRESS • NEW YORK

Published by Three Rivers Press, New York, New York.
Member of the Crown Publishing Group, a division of Random House, Inc.
www.randomhouse.com

THREE RIVERS PRESS and the Tugboat design are registered trademarks of Random House, Inc.

Tom Patire, Hom-Do, Training for Life, and STOP-EM are trademarks owned by Tom Patire. CDT and all other CDT course names like SKYSAFE are trademarks owned by Tom Patire & CDT Training Inc.

Printed in the United States of America

DESIGN BY ELINA D. NUDELMAN

Library of Congress Cataloging-in-Publication Data
Patire, Tom.
    [Personal protection handbook]
    Tom Patire's Personal protection handbook : absolutely everything you need to know to keep yourself, your family, and your assets safe / Tom Patire. — 1st ed.
1. Self-defense.   2. Crime prevention.   I. Title.
GV1111.P37   2003
613.6'6—dc21   2003007699

ISBN 1-4000-4907-5

10 9 8 7 6 5 4 3 2 1

First Edition

IN LOVING MEMORY OF PHILIP AND ELEANOR PATIRE.

AS A CHILD I WATCHED, AS A TEENAGER I LEARNED, AND AS A MAN I KNEW THAT BOTH OF YOU, MOM AND DAD, HAD GIVEN ME EVERY TOOL NEEDED TO LIVE A PROTECTIVE LIFE, AND THAT IT WAS NOW MY TIME TO PUT THEM TO WORK. THOUGH GOD HAS TAKEN YOU FROM US AND LEFT A VOID IN OUR HEARTS, I REALIZE MORE THAN EVER HOW MUCH LOVE AND RESPECT I HAVE FOR BOTH OF YOU. I WILL TRULY MISS YOU, BUT I WILL NEVER FORGET YOU. I AM TRULY PROUD TO BE YOUR SON AND WILL UPHOLD THE HONOR AND INTEGRITY OF THE PATIRE NAME UNTIL IT IS MY TIME TO PASS IT ON.

ACKNOWLEDGMENTS

FIRST AND FOREMOST, thanks to my wife, Doris, and my son, Tommy, who gave me the love, support, and encouragement I needed during the trials and tribulations of writing a book.

Special thanks to my brothers, Phil and Tim, not only for their support but also for protecting their youngest brother all those years until I was ready to protect myself.

My sincere thanks and deepest respect to Alan J. Robinson, Richard Faustini, Mark Prach, and Mel Klein for contributing their expertise as well as for their enduring friendship. Added thanks to my staff, Darren Hamilton, Mat Buonomo, Joe Wyka, Mike Constantino, and Vince Damiano (who also created the line art that appears in the book), as well as to all the CDT instructors and trainees throughout the world who embrace the Training for Life philosophy not as a fad but as a commitment to making the world a safer and more secure place.

Professional thanks to my literary agent, Barbara Lowenstein, who, after seeing me on television, took the initiative to call and motivate me to write this book. And to Judy Kern for her magic in helping bring my words to life and her guidance throughout the process.

Finally, thanks to my dearest friend, Dave Geliebter, who guided me through the unfamiliar waters of business and allowed me freedom of expression while making sure I had the support and foundation to stay afloat in these waters.

CONTENTS

TOM PATIRE'S

PERSONAL
PROTECTION

HANDBOOK

INTRODUCTION

IMMEDIATELY FOLLOWING THE TRAGEDY of September 11, 2001, requests for enrollment in the personal and family protection classes at CDT training centers throughout the world increased at least tenfold. As the world grapples with the question of how to protect innocent civilians from terrorist groups, neighborhood gangs, and individual criminals who are willing to inflict harm, or even kill, in order to achieve their objectives, it becomes more and more impossible to ignore our need to take personal responsibility for our own safety and that of our families. If educating ourselves about personal protection was once an option, it is now, without doubt, a responsibility.

There's certainly nothing wrong with trying to increase airport security or screen people entering public spaces and office buildings, but the fact remains that no security arrangements, no matter how well thought out or implemented, can take the place of personal vigilance. We all need to be alert and prepared for any eventuality as we go about our daily lives. Even a momentary lapse of focus or simple absentmindedness can sometimes make the difference between triumph and tragedy, between walking away unharmed and losing one's life.

Although it is difficult to imagine that anyone, anywhere in the world, is not by this time aware that terrorism can strike anywhere at any time, very few of us, luckily, will ever be the victim of a terrorist act. All of us, however, are vulnerable to any number of much more common life-threatening situations, not all of which are necessarily brought about by a person or persons intending to do us harm.

I CREDIT ONE PARTICULAR incident in my early life with my decision to dedicate myself to protecting others. It occurred when my older brother, Tim, and I were both in high school and Tim was dating a cheerleader who had recently broken up with one of the captains of the football team. Word traveled throughout the school that Patire was dating this guy's girlfriend. The trouble was that "word" didn't include which Patire it was. As I was walking out of class one day, this so-called tough football player pushed me from behind, headfirst into a garbage can, and then, in true bully style, proceeded to punch me while I was down. A couple of teachers broke it up, but I was an emotional and physical mess. My father came to pick me up at the nurse's office, but it wasn't until my brother got home that evening that I found out why I'd been targeted. He was a tough kid and I was his younger brother, and I knew, just looking at him, that he would even the score. And the next day he did. He and two of his friends went to school and met up with the guy who'd hurt me. Tim took care of business while his friends stood by to make sure the fight was fair and that no one intervened.

At the time this occurred, I was still small for my age. In grammar school I was tiny. When I graduated from high school I was skinny and only five feet six. I hated my size, but my mother and my maternal grandmother were always telling me, "Don't worry, Tom, you'll grow." And they were right. In college I grew to six feet three and 225 pounds, and between participating in sports and practicing martial arts, I got myself into top shape. But I never forgot being bullied as a small kid in high school, and when I graduated from William Paterson University with a bachelor of arts degree in Human Movement, I decided to put my education, expertise, and life experience to work.

I have been in the business of protecting other people ever since.

Originally, martial arts was my passion. As a child, I concentrated mainly on aikido, but I also went on to study a variety of traditional styles before discovering that "traditional" was not my cup of tea. So I then learned a combative art called Hom-Do that, in those days, was looked upon as a renegade system, and it fit me like a glove. I guess I've always been something of a renegade at heart because I've never been one to follow in anyone else's footsteps, but have always preferred to do things my own way.

Eventually, doing it my way led me to determine that when it came to personal protection for the average person, brains over brawn was truly the way to go. With that in mind, I developed my own personal system, called CDT (Compliance, Direction, Takedown), based on temporarily disabling rather than annihilating an attacker, which I've now been teaching to many thousands of average citizens as well as protection professionals since 1989.

Traditionally, bodyguarding has followed the Secret Service model, which is extremely effective in certain situations. In the private sector, however, there are often limited resources, limited manpower, and certain budgetary constraints that aren't a concern when the person you're guarding is the president of the United States or some other high-level government official. I started out traveling the conventional protection circuit, establishing my reputation, but whenever I was given the chance, I would demonstrate my own system, and before I knew it, word had spread.

I come from a law-enforcement family. My father was a police officer in Lodi, New Jersey, but, having grown up hearing about the political jungle he had to navigate every day, I never wanted to follow in his footsteps. As my career advanced and my reputation grew, however, I found that various government agencies were swearing me in as a special or auxiliary training officer to get around the fact that I wasn't actually an official member of law enforcement, so that I could teach seminars or hold training sessions in control tactics and weapon disarms at their academies. As time went on, however, it became clear that obtaining certification was essential to teaching law-enforcement personnel, so I went through certification courses such as the FBI Tactics Instructor Course, which I attended at Fort Dix, New Jersey, so that I could be approved to teach. But even in those courses I was often given the honor of being asked to demonstrate my own version of controlling or take-out tactics. Today many of the agencies I went to for certification send their people to my courses for theirs.

Eventually my reputation spread even farther, and I was asked to travel to other countries, including Denmark, Peru, Mexico, and the Philippines, as a private consultant, helping to develop tactical courses for their law-enforcement, military, and security agencies. Adapting to foreign customs and fitting into hostile environments were certainly new challenges, but I took them head-on and, happily, did very well.

AS A PROFESSIONAL BODYGUARD, I've been involved in my share of life-or-death situations, and I've witnessed more than a few terrible events. But I've always been able to separate my emotions from my job and do what needed to be done—until I got my own "wake-up call." My first visceral realization of how vulnerable all of us are as human beings occurred several years before the attack on the World Trade Center, when my wife, Doris, and I lost our first child at birth and she then, during her second pregnancy, developed an illness that threatened to take her life as well as that of our unborn child. Thankfully, both my wife and my son are now thriving and healthy, but that near-tragedy really brought home to me, very personally, how much of life is totally beyond our control.

As a husband and father with an extremely busy work schedule, I also came to realize that there are many times when it's simply not possible for me to be there watching over my loved ones—even though, as a protection professional and something of a control freak, I'd certainly like to do that. At least in this regard, I know that I'm no different from millions of other people throughout this country and around the world. And it was that realization which gave me the impetus to write this book.

I have made it my mission, both in my courses and in my writing, to use my training and knowledge to teach as many ordinary people as I can—men, women, and even children—not only about their responsibility to protect themselves and their families, but also about the simple and practical techniques they can learn to use on an everyday basis. My work has given me access to the minds and experience of a variety of law-enforcement officials, and to the "expertise" of many professional criminals. As part of my research, I've written to and interviewed inmates, former inmates, and men on work-release programs at the Allenwood Correctional Institute in Allenwood, Pennsylvania, and at the Bergen County Jail and the Morris County Jail in New Jersey. These men have provided me with eye-opening insights into the criminal mind. I've used the "insider" knowledge I've gained from both sides of the law to make this book both comprehensive and practical in real-life situations.

I don't encourage anyone to take risks for the sake of simple heroics. I know all too well that most of our heroes are dead. And I don't teach combative martial arts as the answer for everyone. I'm aware that in the heat of the very real moment, what we've learned under controlled circumstances in the gym or a martial-arts training center more often than not will desert us because, although our bodies are conditioned, our minds are not prepared. A seasoned martial artist would, in my opinion, do well in an altercation as long as his training was realistic and he'd had some previous experience with an opponent. Most of us, when we're under extreme stress or when we're afraid, whether or not we think we're going to be able to "keep our heads," will be thrown into a state commonly known as "fight or flight" when our autonomic (or involuntary) nervous system kicks in. When that happens, our bloodstream is flooded with adrenaline, our vision and hearing are affected, the mind fills with a sea of emotions, and we simply can't think as clearly as we do normally.

The goal of my training is to allow people under extreme stress to respond automatically, using simple, practiced actions so that even if their conscious thought process shuts down, their bodies will still know what to do because the training will be embedded in muscle memory. My intent is to allow good people to walk away from bad situations with little or no injury, and, in the case of a personal attack, to disable their attacker using nondeadly force. I don't want to turn mommies into Charlie's Angels or daddies into ninjas, but I do want to give them the ability to protect their own lives and families in situations where there is no alternative. I don't teach violence; I teach people how to avoid or, when necessary, to escape acts of violence.

The methods I teach result from years of research and have been proved effective over and over again. They involve practicing awareness and mastering trained responses. Just as it's a lot easier for an actor to work from a memorized script than to improvise each time he goes onstage, so it is easier and certainly more effective for us to respond to the unexpected with simple, scripted movements and rehearsed actions than to react "off the cuff." When we react in the heat of the moment without training or planning, we're likely to do more harm than good, and too often it's not the "bad guys" but ourselves and our families who are harmed.

Just this year, a single mom came to me with her twelve-year-old son to learn some techniques for defending both of them. She explained that she lived on a limited income because she had no real skills and no formal education. Her son, she told me, was the only thing she had that meant anything to her.

During the first week of their training, I taught her nothing more than how to move herself in front of her child and talk into the attacker's direct line of sight, allowing him to concentrate on her so that her child could escape to safety. The theory behind this tactic is that if the child is out of sight, he will also be out of the mind of the bad guy and one less thing for the mother to worry about if she needs to defend herself or escape. When the mother practiced distraction, the child eased his way to safety and called attention to himself by screaming, just as I'd taught him. I could see from the way these two worked together that there was a genuine love between them and that they made a very good team.

Unfortunately, it wasn't too long before this mother and son got the opportunity to put their newly learned skills to the test. On Halloween night they were on their way home from the library when they were confronted by a guy in a scary mask. He asked the woman for her money, and when she told him she didn't have any, he asked for her son. At that point she stepped in front of the boy and yelled, "Don't touch my child." That was the signal the child had learned in training, which meant it was time for him to take off, yelling, "Help, help, they're hurting my mother," and that's exactly what he did.

Within seconds, two construction workers heard the child screaming and saw him running down the sidewalk. When they looked around and saw the mother running from a masked man, they tackled the man. One held him down while the other called the police, who arrived on the scene and arrested him.

As it turned out, the man was a neighbor who wanted money for drugs. When the woman told him she didn't have any, he thought he'd take her son and hold him for ransom. The key to the success of this story was the love between the two intended victims, which, in this case, was reinforced by their best ally—realistic, proven training that combines movement and verbal distraction but requires absolutely no violence.

THREE REASONS THINGS GO WRONG

The Bad Guest

When I address groups of people about the need to take responsibility for personal protection, I explain that there are three types of threats we need to fear, or three reasons things can go wrong. The first, and statistically the most frequent, I call the Bad Guest. A Bad Guest is someone we know or with whom we've had some kind of friendly contact, who, for whatever reason, takes advantage of us. Situations involving a Bad Guest include domestic violence, date rape, or simply theft of money that happens to be lying around in a visible or accessible location. The crime could be fueled by alcohol or drugs or simply by opportunism.

The Bad Guest phenomenon begins to play a role as early as childhood, when kids get together and someone in the group is a bit more rambunctious or mischievous than the others. Then, as children become teenagers, the Bad Guest might be the pushy guy who wants a little something more than a kiss from his girlfriend or wants to instigate trouble among his peers. In adulthood, the Bad Guest is the one who pushes the envelope either with you or someone else in your home or your group, creating what I call situational violence.

I saw how this can happen when a friend asked me to go with him to watch his little boy play in a league championship baseball game for six-to-eight-year-olds. Needless to say, the stands were packed with parents cheering for their little ones. In the bottom of the seventh inning, the score was tied. My friend's son's team was in the field and their opponents had a man on third with one out. The next kid up hit a ball down the third-base line that appeared to be foul. The umpire, however, called it fair. The kid on third scored and the team went on to win the championship.

When that happened, one of the parents ran out onto the field and started berating the umpire who'd made the call. As the ump tried to explain what he'd seen, the irate father just got more and more worked up. When a second umpire came over to try to mediate the situation, the father lit into him, too. Meanwhile, all the kids just stood around watching. My friend went out onto the field to grab his son, and, just as he did, the now-incensed father punched one of the umpires, a man in his sixties, in the face. The umpire's son, who happened to be in the stands that day, then came out and grabbed his father's assailant, hitting him in the face and knocking him to the ground.

Right about then the police showed up and arrested both the umpire's son and the man who had started the fight. Both teams had been invited for pizza at the local VFW hall after the big game, but the only thing any of those kids could talk about was the "cool" fight. Not one of them mentioned winning the championship or the fun they'd had playing the game.

HOW TO SPOT A BAD GUEST IN A CROWD

- Look for the person who seems either preoccupied or agitated.
- Listen for *what* the person is saying and *how* they are saying it.
- Listen for abrupt changes in tone of voice. Does it become either louder or unnaturally quiet?
- Watch for changes in facial expression. Does it become nastier or show increasing signs of stress? Or does the person look dazed and show no expression at all?
- Look for changes in the eyes. Are they becoming narrower? Darting about?
- Watch for aggressive hand movements accompanying verbal outbursts.
- Look for any behavior that seems inappropriate for the given situation—too loud, too quiet, not participating or interacting with others.

TOM'S TIP

Like that father, many Bad Guests are, for the most part, decent human beings who, for one reason or another, get the wrong button pushed one day and act badly. For most it's a one-time offense, and once it's all over, they are careful to watch themselves in the future.

The Bad Guy

The second type of threat comes from the Bad Guy, a seasoned criminal for whom crime is a business. The harm might be either physical or material (theft of property), but it is instigated by someone with a criminal mindset.

Bad Guys feed off wreaking havoc with your body and mind, and will stop at nothing to achieve their goal. They may be bad, but they're also smart, and they know that most "good" people are untrained and unsure of themselves when it comes to personal

BAD GUEST/BAD GUY:
YOUR ODDS OF BECOMING A VICTIM

The National Crime Victimization Survey reports that in 2001, United States residents aged 12 or over experienced a total of 24.2 million crimes, broken down as follows:

- ➡ 76 % (18.3 million) crimes against property
- ➡ 24% (5.7 million) crimes of violence
- ➡ 2% personal theft

In that same year, for every 1,000 persons aged 12 or older, there occurred

- ➡ 1 rape or sexual assault
- ➡ 2 assaults with injury
- ➡ 3 robberies

protection. If you become the target of a Bad Guy, it's probably because you've made yourself a target by bragging in public about something you had of value, or by appearing to be preoccupied and oblivious of your surroundings rather than alert and aware of what's going on around you.

The latter is exactly what happened to two sisters in their mid-fifties who lived together in an older house surrounded by shrubbery at the end of a one-way street. The two women did everything together, including working at the same department store. One day in December they both took off from work to go holiday shopping. Preoccupied with what they were doing, they were unaware that they'd been targeted and were being followed by a pair of teenage hoodlums.

At about six o'clock in the evening they stopped at a local coffee shop for a bite to eat, again absorbed in discussing their day and talking about how much wrapping they'd have to do. When they left the coffee shop about an hour later, they were again followed by the same group of teens.

Once they pulled into their driveway and the teenagers saw that it was obscured by bushes and that many of the outside lights had burned out and never been replaced, they made their way around to the back, where the ladies were unloading their car. They yanked the women by the hair, pushed them to the ground, and then grabbed them by their throats. One of them demanded the car keys and directed the terrified victims to crawl under a table on their patio and commanded them not to move. He then drove off in their car while his pal drove off in his, not realizing that they were going the wrong way on a one-way street. As the first car got to the cross street, it was spotted by a police officer, who gave chase. The first kid was apprehended not ten blocks from where the robbery took place, and within a few hours he gave up his partner as well.

HOW TO SPOT A BAD GUY

Since Bad Guys are often professionals, they are admittedly often harder to spot than Bad Guests. There are, however, a few overt signs to look out for:

- Inappropriate dress. Wearing a long coat on a hot day, for example, could mean a Bad Guy is concealing a weapon.

- Inappropriate actions, such as standing on the sidelines and not participating in the activity going on around him.

- Inappropriate facial expression, such as a blank stare when everyone else is smiling.

- Unfocused eyes, edginess, or profuse sweating while standing still; these might indicate drug use or intoxication.

TOM'S TIP

When the police returned the women's car and their possessions, the victims couldn't stop talking about how shocked they were at having been targeted and followed.

The Bad Day

Finally, and statistically least likely, is the Bad Day, which might mean simply that we're going about our ordinary business when a total stranger just snaps and takes out his or her frustrations on us. Or, in the worst-case scenario, we might fall victim to a catastrophic event such as that of September 11, one that has global consequences not only in loss of life but also in terms of the financial disaster that follows in its aftermath. A Bad Day is when we're going about our business as usual and the worst of the worst, the fear of all fears, enters our world.

Even before September 11, I'd been contacted by various airline personnel who'd been involved in violent airborne situations that had caused them serious injury, hospitalization, and many months out of work. In response to these requests, I have designed a unique training course called SKYSAFE, which provides flight attendants and frequent flyers with the skills they need to level the playing field and improve their chances of escaping uninjured from what might otherwise have turned into a very Bad Day.

TERRORISM AND EXTREMISM

Terrorism and extremism have been with us virtually since the beginning of time. Defining terrorism, however, is not as easy as it used to be. The United States Department of Justice and the State Department define terrorism as "the unlawful use of—or threatened use of—force or violence, in violation of the accepted rules of warfare, and a sovereign nation's laws, during a time of peace or conflict, against individuals or property to coerce or intimidate governments, societies or individuals, intended to achieve political, religious or ideological objectives."

Acts of terrorism during the 1980s and 1990s were most often

THE ODDS OF HAVING A BAD DAY
ON THE GROUND OR IN THE AIR

The Fatality Analysis Reporting System statistics indicate that:

- In 2001 (the most recent year for which statistics are available) there were 37,795 vehicular fatalities, 269 more than in the previous year. This averages to 1.5 fatalities for each 100 million vehicle miles traveled.

- The most recent information on train travel indicates that between January and June of 2002 there were a total of 6,708 accidents, resulting in 468 fatalities.

- According to planecrashinfo.com, there have been 2,125 accidents involving commercial aircraft between 1950 and 2001.

- If you flew the 25 airlines with the best safety records, your odds of being involved in an airline fatality would be 1 in 3.72 million.

state-sponsored. Libya, for example, was a major sponsor or supporter of terrorism until it was bombed by the United States during the Reagan administration. Today, while there continue to be a few state sponsors, many terrorist acts are carried out by loosely formed groups of people such as Hamas in the Middle East, the ETA in Spain, the MLF in the Philippines, and Al Qaeda. These groups are harder to track and identify because they have several layers of leadership and no central physical base of operations.

Another recent development in the world of terrorism is the rise of the so-called "Ozzie and Harriet" terrorist, people like Timothy McVeigh, who work alone or with only one or two others and who blend into the population, maybe even have children on the soccer team, but who are disgruntled about issues like abortion, animal rights, globalization, or the environment, or are angry at their own government for one reason or another. Their extremist views can eventually culminate in an act of violence or terrorism.

There are also apparently normal but disturbed people who are one step away from divorce or from bankruptcy or who have lost their jobs and seek revenge in a very deadly manner. These are the kinds of people whom you see on *America's Most Wanted,* but who are not considered terrorists by the U.S. government.

Unfortunately, terrorism and extremism are here to stay. The more you know about them and prepare yourself and your family, the safer you will be.

I would like to thank Steven J. Fustero, President of the IACSP (International Association for Counterterrorism and Security Professionals) for sharing his expertise on this subject. You can find more information by logging on to his website, www.iacsp.com. The U.S. government also has many articles and updates on their websites, www.fbi.gov, www.whitehouse.gov, www.usdoj.gov, www.dod.gov, www.fema.gov.

Biological or Chemical Attacks

When I appeared on *Good Day New York* as a security expert to talk about what to do in case of a terrorist strike, the hosts of the show, Jim Ryan, Lyn Brown, and Dave Price, spoke for the majority of New Yorkers as well as people throughout the country when they asked me to address the issue of a possible chemical or biological attack.

I explained that, while I don't consider myself an expert on bioterrorism, I have made it my business to educate myself about how to detect the presence of chemical or biological substances and how best to protect myself from them. First, one must understand that it is called bioterrorism because these weapons are designed to strike terror into the hearts and minds of their intended victims. The reason that so much attention has been focused on highly populated, enclosed areas such as office buildings or subways is that an attack in such a venue is most likely to affect a large number of people and to cause mass panic and hysteria.

The best way to protect oneself is to be aware of what to look for. One telltale sign would be an odor not normally associated with its location, such as a sweet, fruity, or fresh-cut-grass smell in the subway. Any kind of suspicious or unusual fire might indicate that chemicals are being burned and releasing toxic fumes. Brown syrupy substances might indicate the presence of other forms of poisonous agents. Physical symptoms of exposure to toxins might be coughing, difficulty in breathing, a runny nose, nausea, or tightness in the chest, to name just a few.

While the police and other first responders have undergone and continue to receive extensive training in how to detect and respond to these kinds of attacks, we must also understand that they are, by definition, responding after the fact, and that there is no way of knowing how much time might elapse between the attack and the response. In light of that knowledge, we would all do best to hone our self-preservation skills so that we can act as first responders for ourselves.

CHECKLIST FOR SURVIVING A BIOLOGICAL OR CHEMICAL ATTACK

✔ *Read the environment.* Do you detect an unusual odor, even if it isn't unpleasant? Are people around you getting sick? Think "What is wrong with this picture?"

✔ *Remain calm.* Try to remain rational, consider what you need to do to survive, and deal with the moment.

✔ *Control your breathing.* Not only will this help to control your anxiety, but the better able you are to control your breathing, the less toxic substance is likely to enter your lungs.

✔ *Think before you move.* Pause to determine the quickest and safest route to the most accessible exit, then move deliberately toward it. If you're in an enclosed environment, your goal is to reach the open air as quickly as possible.

✔ *Check your person.* If you see or feel the presence of any substance that is burning or blistering your skin, blot it off with whatever disposal substance is immediately accessible. Do not rub the spot; this is likely to spread rather than contain the toxin and cause even more irritation.

✔ *Believe in yourself.* Remember that to survive this kind of attack you need to think, act, and follow your plan.

A FOURTH REASON THINGS GO WRONG:
BAD JUDGMENT

In addition to the Bad Guest, Bad Guy, and Bad Day scenarios, there are also situations in which simple lack of forethought, or not taking into account the possible risks attendant on an everyday act, might turn out to have harmful consequences.

Not too long ago, I was told about a potentially serious accident that occurred when a young woman was driving her car and drinking a bottle of iced tea on her way to pick up a friend to go to the local shopping mall. She arrived at her destination and honked her horn. Her friend said she'd be out in a few minutes, so the young woman finished her tea and stashed the empty bottle on the passenger side of the dashboard. Her friend came out and they went on their way. While they were on the highway, chatting and listening to the radio, a truck stopped short in front of them. The young woman driving stomped on the brake and skidded to a halt, causing the empty iced-tea bottle to catapult off the dashboard, hitting the passenger in the face. Luckily she suffered nothing more than a sizable lump on her forehead, but that same bottle could have shattered or hit her on the nose or the eye instead of the forehead, causing much more serious damage.

Taking responsibility for our personal safety—and that of our family and friends—means more than simply being alert to obviously dangerous situations or potential criminal threats. It also means being more conscious at all times of the harm that could come from even the most innocent of everyday accidents.

HOW TO USE THIS BOOK

I've used the methods in this book to train tens of thousands of women and men in CDT centers throughout the country, and now I hope to reach thousands more of you who, for whatever reason, can't come to a center to learn them one-on-one, so that you, too, will have opened your eyes and your minds in order to live a safer, more secure life.

PAY ATTENTION TO DETAILS

The little things in life can make a big difference. Body and mind are an unbeatable team as long as you are focusing on the moment and thinking about safety. Too many of us are preoccupied—talking on a cell phone when we should be concentrating on driving, rushing from one place to another without scanning our surroundings or watching where and how we walk.

When we're not paying attention and our mind isn't on what we're doing, even everyday tasks like cooking, walking outside to get the mail, or just playing with our kids in the house can lead to life-altering accidents.

TOM'S TIP

To get the most out of this information, you should first read it straight through from beginning to end. Going directly to the physical techniques in chapter six, or skipping any section, will mean that you've left out one or more pieces of the puzzle that have been designed to fit together in a particular order. I'm a methodical guy—in my line of work I have to be—and I've thought through and laid out this material in the best and easiest way for the greatest number of people to absorb and put into action.

If you're tempted to skip the section on protecting your family, for example, because you're single and have no children, stop and consider whether you might, at some time, be in a situation where a child in your company, or the child of someone you're close to, was threatened. Wouldn't you want to be prepared to come to the child's aid or offer your assistance? None of us lives in isolation, and it's impossible to know when even the most unexpected situation might arise. I urge you, therefore, at least to look through every section and think about when or how the information it contains might—just might—become useful for you.

In the final chapter you'll find the five essential moves I teach in my basic CDT classes, or what I now call the Training for Life program. They are physical maneuvers based on everyday motions like knocking on a door or turning a key, and they are all easy to perform, whether you're big or small, young or old, male or female. Each of the five moves is fully illustrated and is based on the theory that the hands do the motion, but the mind gives you the process. As you work through this book, the reasoning behind that theory will become clear—and that's another reason why it's so important that you begin at the beginning and read through to the end.

For now, however, what you need to know is that you're holding in your hands a complete program for personal protection that starts with training your mind. After you train your mind, you'll be better equipped to train your body.

ONE

DON'T BE A VICTIM

A WELL-DRESSED WOMAN *shopping at a local mall one afternoon was quietly being targeted by a savvy pair of thieves who, having identified her as a person of means, were following her on her rounds, trailing her from one shop to the next.*

When her hands were full of shopping bags as she returned to her car, which was parked in the enclosed garage, they saw the opportunity to make their move. They waited until she was backing out of her space and bumped her car with their van, just hard enough to cause her to stop and get out to inspect the damage. At that point they grabbed her, put a knife to her throat, and threw her into the back of the van, where they robbed her of more than $1,000 in purchases, $500 in cash, and all the jewelry she was wearing, including her wedding ring.

And then, because she made the foolish mistake of talking back to them instead of keeping quiet, they had the last word by pouring a cup of cold coffee over her head and forcing her to lie on the floor of the garage while they made their getaway. When the police arrived, the first thing she did was to berate them for not being there when she needed them.

Later that evening she called me in to track down the robbers, which turned out to be virtually impossible, since she was unable to furnish any identifying information about either her assailants or the van.

○ ○ ○

THERE ARE SEVERAL LESSONS to be learned from this cautionary tale. The first and probably the most important is that no one should ever consider himself or herself immune from this kind of attack. My client, as she told me, had felt she was "safe" because she was relatively affluent and wasn't traveling in the kind of neighborhood where she'd expect a robbery to take place. Her misapprehension is all too common, but my answer is simply this: If you were to think about robbing someone, would you do it in a place where your victim was unlikely to have much money, or would you go someplace where you'd be more likely to find a person carrying cash and wearing valuable jewelry?

Second, when you're out shopping, wherever it is, dress unobtrusively, don't wear flashy jewelry, and be aware of your surroundings. Had this woman been more vigilant, she might well have spotted her would-be assailants before they had the chance to accost her in the garage. Had she not been so clearly a person with money—as signaled by her jewelry and clothing, not to mention the amount of money she was obviously spending—they might have chosen someone else. And had she sent them a message through her body language that she was alert to what was going on around her, she might have made herself a less attractive target.

Finally, if you do have the misfortune to be the victim of a robbery, keep your eyes open and your mouth shut. There's nothing really to be gained from verbally "dissing" your attackers, and, as was the case with this woman, you might just get them angry enough to want to humiliate or harm you further. In any dangerous situation, your main goal should be to escape unharmed, not giving the bad guys a piece of your mind. And, as my client later confessed, she was silly enough to be more concerned about preserving her freshly manicured nails than about memorizing a description of the thieves or their van, thus rendering herself totally useless as a source of information, to either the police who responded to her call or to me.

CHECKLIST FOR CONFRONTATION

✔ *Concentrate on the positive.* Think about what you can do, not what might be done to you. Remaining proactive might just prevent you from suffering even further harm. Feeling sorry for yourself or falling prey to self-doubt isn't going to help you. Instead, listen, follow directions, and watch what you say as well as how you say it. All situations, no matter how desperate, provide a window of opportunity for survival or escape. You need to buy yourself time and be alert to that opportunity when it comes.

✔ *Focus on the moment.* The danger is that fear will prevent you from thinking clearly. Physiologically, fear causes the nervous system to send adrenaline rushing to the brain, putting us into panic, or what is commonly known as fight-or-flight mode. The resulting neurological changes can affect our vision, our hearing, and our ability to think clearly.

✔ *Review the situation in your mind.* You need to be prepared to assess all your options quickly, to ensure that your response will be the one most likely to get you out of the situation unharmed.

✔ *Act, don't react.* This goes along with remaining proactive and taking the initiative, rather than allowing the criminal to be the one who "calls the shots." Expect the unexpected by being aware and prepared.

✔ *When in doubt, ease your way out.* My philosophy has always been that there's no point in being a hero if you're going to be a dead hero. And there's no shame in making self-protection your number-one goal—even if that means letting the bad guys get away. There's nothing more valuable than life itself. In any potentially life-threatening situation, preserving your material possessions must come second to preserving your life.

✔ *Whenever possible, use verbal rather than physical skills.* Unless you're extremely well trained, extremely skilled, and absolutely certain you can come out of the situation unscathed, getting physical with an attacker can really get you hurt. That doesn't mean, however, that you should taunt your attacker, thereby adding fuel to his fire; your words should be aimed at dousing the flames, not inflaming his anger.

HOW TO TALK TO A BAD GUY

- Tone of voice can make all the difference. Keep it calm and consistent.

- Never talk down to the bad guy, and don't attempt the approach that suggests you try to make him your ally by convincing him you "want to help." He won't buy it. Would you?

- Listen carefully and respond directly to questions. For example, if he asks, "Where is the cash?," don't reply, "The jewelry is in my top drawer."

- Stay focused and attentive at all times. Keep your wits about you.

- Don't make statements that could make the situation worse. For example, "I don't want any problems; I am not going to give you a hard time" is okay. But saying "I'll do whatever you want" could lead from a robbery to a rape.

- Pay attention, speak only when spoken to, and be attentive to his movements.

- Make sure you stress that you don't want to create a problem.

TOM'S TIP

✔ *Trust in yourself and follow your instincts.* Again, this goes along with keeping your mind focused and responding rather than reacting. We all have an internal alarm system; when yours goes off, trust your gut and do what it's telling you to do.

✔ *Remember that trained movement is almost always more effective than irrational behavior.* That's what this book is all about. It will give you the edge you need to survive in any situation that threatens you or your family.

In the chapters that follow, I'll be providing you with the specific tools you'll need to begin your own Training for Life, which means training not only your body but also your mind so that you'll be prepared to use the eight steps above in order to give yourself a chance to survive in any confrontation.

WHO IS THE MOST LIKELY VICTIM?

In researching this book, I spoke with many different people—victims and victimizers alike—and I discovered that there were, in fact, patterns of behavior that would make one more or less attractive as a target for criminal attack.

One thing I learned is that, psychologically, many people are unwilling to contemplate even the possibility that they might ever be targeted for a criminal act. They prefer to adhere to the "out of sight, out of mind" mentality, and therefore they simply don't take the proactive steps that might help to ensure their own safety and the safety of their loved ones.

The people I spoke with who had been victims reacted in one of two ways. Many "good" people were so incredulous that such a bad thing could have happened to them that they were incapable of moving past their sense of having been "wronged" to take the steps that would prevent the same thing from happening again. Others, however, admitted that the attack occurred at a time when they were too preoccupied to remain focused on what they were doing at the moment, and that their lapse in concentration had created the opportunity for the crime. The people in this second group are the ones who are more likely to make sure they do things differently the next time, and who are less likely to make the same mistake again. My goal is to help you learn how to do things right the first time, before it becomes necessary for you to learn from unfortunate experience.

The criminals with whom I spoke or corresponded gave me great information about what might make someone a victim. Their rationale for choosing a target was not so much "Why victimize this person?" as "Why not victimize this person?" The victim, in other words, more often than not, offers himself up as a target by appearing distracted, disorganized, and unfocused. Or, as one seasoned criminal put it, "We don't pick our victims. They pick themselves."

Criminals look upon our misfortune as their good fortune. They are really opportunists who look upon crime as a business, and their goal is to make the most profit with the least risk and effort. Mainly, they want to minimize their exposure to the possibility of being caught. And, like most businessmen, those who are the most successful are the best at what they do. If a "business" opportunity presents itself to someone with a criminal mind, you can be sure that he'll be ready and willing to capitalize on the prospect. And those who consistently offer the greatest opportunity for profit with the least potential risk are, as you might expect, women, children, and the elderly.

THE FEMALE TARGET

As a group, women are the most frequent crime victims. Women alone may certainly be attractive targets for mugging or robbery simply because they're smaller and, at least in theory, weaker than men and also less likely to "fight back." But the kinds of attacks women fear most are domestic violence and rape.

Domestic Violence

The American Medical Association estimates that more than 4 million women every year become victims of severe domestic violence by male companions. Approximately one in every four women is likely to be abused by an intimate companion at some time in her life.

At our Training for Life events I always ask, "How many people here have ever experienced some form of domestic violence?" Almost invariably, more than half of the 500 or more attendees raise their hands. My next question is usually, "How many of you did not report it to the authorities?" More than 75 percent of those who raised their hands the first time raise them again, which indicates that the AMA's estimates are probably much too low.

HOW TO GET HELP

Many incidents of domestic violence go unreported because women are afraid or don't know where to go for help.

The National Domestic Violence Hotline, 1-800-799-SAFE or 1-800-787-3224, is the place to call. It is open twenty-four hours a day, 365 days a year; it maintains a database of more than 4,000 shelters and service providers across the United States; it keeps all calls strictly confidential; and it has answered more than 700,000 phone calls from victims of domestic violence since its inception.

TOM'S TIP

After these events, many of the women who have suffered domestic violence come up to speak with me privately. Their reasons for not reporting these incidents range from fear of retaliation to still "having feelings" for their abuser.

The FBI's Uniform Crime Reports states that 85 percent of all domestic violence reports involve female victims, and that 64 percent of those females are white.

Rape

The best ways to avoid the threat of rape should be fairly obvious. Keep away from isolated areas; stay on main roadways and well-lit streets; be alert to your surroundings; and be selective in choosing the people with whom you fraternize. But if you do fall victim to a rape, it's important to keep your wits about you. Don't expend all your energy on futile attempts to escape. Wait for your best moment—such as when your attacker is using his hands to pull down his pants—and then use your self-defense training, if you have any, or just hit (or kick) and run. (The five CDT moves in chapter six are also highly valuable in the event of a sexual assault.) If there's more than one attacker, or if your assailant is armed, the situation becomes both more difficult and more dangerous, and, again, it's most important to try to remain clear-headed. Is there anything nearby you can use as a weapon? Would it be better to appear to cooperate while you await your best opportunity for escape? By training your senses, as I'll be explaining in the chapters that follow, you'll be more likely to use them to your advantage in even the most frightening of circumstances.

If the rapist is a complete stranger, he's certainly a Bad Guy, but all too often a rapist can be a Bad Guest. According to the National Crime Victimization Survey completed in 2000, approximately 62 percent of rape victims know their assailants. Those at highest risk are white women between the ages of twelve and thirty-four. Sex Offenses and Offenders lists the average age of the rapist as approximately thirty-one.

Like incidents of domestic violence, many rapes are unreported for a variety of reasons. When I ask at a Training for Life event, "Why would someone not report a rape?" the reason most commonly given is that the victim didn't want to go though the court system and experience things she had seen in movies or on Court TV. Many women said they'd rather live with the nightmare than experience it all over again. And many indicated that their rapist had not been a scary stranger wearing a mask and hiding in a dark alley or the bushes, but someone they knew. Still others reported that their guard had been down because they were in some kind of comfort zone at the time of the attack.

Not too long ago, I spoke to a group of more than 500 women, aged twelve to eighty, on the subject of personal protection. Following my talk, members of the audience came forward to ask me questions, many of which were related to actual events in their lives, usually involving either domestic violence or robbery.

After everyone else had left and I was leaving the building, a young woman who appeared to be about thirty years old came out one of the side doors and asked if she could speak with me alone. I asked my staff to wait, and stepped aside so that we wouldn't be overheard. The woman didn't give her name, but said she'd enjoyed my talk and told me the reason she'd come was that, a year before, she'd been raped repeatedly for a two-hour period by someone she knew.

She told me she'd befriended a man who was very soft-spoken and shy and appeared to be "afraid of his own shadow." After they'd met several times in a local park, he invited her to his apartment, which was not far away. At first she refused, but he made her feel so guilty, saying that he had no friends, that she finally agreed.

Once they got to the apartment, they talked for a while, and when she got up to go to the bathroom he apparently locked all the doors and all the windows and put on the radio and air conditioners to muffle any sound. When she came out, he threw her on the floor and tore off her clothes. He grabbed her by the mouth and told her that if she screamed he'd choke her to death. He raped her three times over the course of the next two hours, promising that if she cooperated he wouldn't kill her. When she started crying, he smacked her in the face until she stopped, and then continued to violate her.

When I asked why she hadn't fought back, she said she'd been too scared. When I asked if she'd had any training, she said she'd taken a martial arts course for three weeks many years before, but had hated it so much that she quit.

She told me the rapist had gone through many mood swings. He was happy, then sad, he laughed, he cried, he was violent and then became gentle. During our conversation she repeated several times that she'd known the guy was unstable and had just hoped he'd let her go when he'd finished with her. Halfway through the ordeal he started to drink, to the point where his words became slurred and his actions sloppy. At some point he dragged her into the living room and turned on the television. From there she could see the front door, and when he got up to refill his glass, she pushed him and ran out of the house.

She never pressed charges because, she said, she didn't want to go through the embarrassment or the mental trauma of reliving the incident. She never saw the man again, and, according to her, she lives her life by thinking of the good and not of the bad. She came to the Training for Life event because she was tired of being paranoid and feeling sorry for herself, and she wanted to do something that would help her take charge of her own life. By attending my seminar she was not only taking her first step toward learning about personal protection, but was also telling someone for the first time the secret she had, until then, been afraid or unwilling to share. She has since taken one of my personal-protection courses and says she now feels empowered and prepared rather than timid and scared.

Stalking

After a course I taught at the Learning Annex in New York City, a woman in her thirties approached to ask if I knew anything about stalkers. When I told her I'd worked several protection details for both celebrities and ordinary citizens who had been the victims of stalkers, she told me that her former boyfriend had become a stalker after they broke up. He would show up at her gym, at her workplace, and at the clubs or restaurants she went to in the evening. One night, after being out of town, she arrived home late at night to find him on her doorstep. She told him she was sick of his turning up everywhere she went, and that he needed to get on with his life. Then she opened the door and let herself into her apartment. A few minutes later she was in the kitchen making a cup of tea, when her boyfriend crashed through the door and grabbed her by the throat, screaming that if he couldn't have her, nobody would. Luckily he yelled so loudly that a neighbor heard him and arrived in time to pull him off her. After a short struggle, the boyfriend ran out the door. The neighbor called the police, the woman filed charges, and the boyfriend was arrested on charges of breaking and entering and assault with intent. When I asked the young woman if that incident was what had brought her to my class, she looked me straight in the eye and said, emphatically, "Yes!"

You don't have to be a celebrity to become a stalking victim.

WHEN YOU'RE STALKED BY AN "EX"

- *Make it obvious it's over:* Be clear that the relationship is history. Show no pity or remorse; to do that gives the stalker a glimmer of hope that "things might work out."

- *Tell everyone:* Make sure the people close to you and to him know that the relationship is over. The more people you tell, the better he will understand that it's over.

- *Make it legal:* Notify the police. If the behavior persists or escalates, file a harassment complaint.

- *Obtain a restraining order:* Use the system that's there to protect you. You need to realize that the person you once cared for has become obsessive, is not thinking clearly, and could be dangerous.

- *Get a big dog:* Especially if you live alone, invest in some type of deterrent, whether it's a dog, an alarm system, or new locks on the doors.

- *Create a check-in system:* Make sure that someone you trust knows where you are at all times, and designate an exact time when you will call that person each day.

- *Be attentive at all times:* Always be aware of your surroundings.

- *Learn personal protection techniques:* The CDT techniques in chapter six could prove invaluable should you face a confrontation.

TOM'S TIP

American Institute of Justice statistics indicate that 8 percent of American women (and 2 percent of men) will be stalked at some time in their lives. The majority of stalkers are men, and the majority of their targets are women.

I categorize stalkers into two groups: the I Group, who have been intimate with and know their intended victims; and the O Group, who are outsiders who have never had personal relationships with their targets. Those in the I Group can't let go. They refuse to accept that the relationship is over. Where the victim can go wrong with this kind of stalker is by showing him sympathy and thus allowing him to believe that there is still some kind of bond between them. The greatest number of stalkers belong in this category.

A typical member of the O Group believes that his victim was meant to be his ideal mate or friend. Even though they've never met, the stalker has created a relationship in his mind that, to him, is very real. Celebrities are most likely to become the victims of this group. Though their behavior may initially be more annoying than dangerous or criminal, it can, and often does, escalate at least to the level of criminal harassment.

THE CHILD TARGET

The children most often targeted for a crime are those unsupervised by adults who, therefore, innocently wander into the wrong place at the wrong time. This is particularly true in apparently safe locations such as busy supermarkets or other large stores. We're more likely to watch our children carefully when they're in a playground, near water, or in other places where we know they can be hurt. But when we're shopping we're more likely to be distracted by the task at hand—whether it's buying groceries or trying on a new outfit. Those who wish to harm children know where to find their best opportunities: exactly the places where parents may be least likely to keep an eye on their children at all times.

One near-tragic incident occurred when the mother of a nine-year-old girl was shopping at her local super store. The woman was moving through the aisles as usual while her daughter straggled behind, stopping to examine and touch whatever caught her eye.

The mother wasn't doing anything out of the ordinary or being particularly negligent. In fact, the same scenario takes place time after time, day after day, in stores throughout the country. So many of us are so pressed for time and thinking about so many things that our minds are seldom in the moment. On this occasion, however, the little girl was approached by a soft-spoken white male who appeared to be in his early fifties. He told her he had a niece about her age and struck up a conversation about a display of rubber balls in different colors, asking her which color was her favorite. When she told him it was red, he took a red ball off the shelf and handed it to her, saying that he was going to buy two, one for her and one for his niece. Then he told her to go with him to the cashier so that he could pay for it. As they walked, he bypassed the register and made his way to the exit with the little girl one step behind. When he got to the door, he put down the second ball he'd been carrying and stuck out his hand for the little girl to grab. When she asked why he hadn't paid for the ball, he just smiled and again reached his hand out. One of the cashiers recognized the little girl from other occasions when she'd been there with her mother, and asked her who the man was. At that point he bolted from the store into a car that was waiting in front with a driver in it and the engine running. The cashier ran out and tried to get the license plate number, but by then the car was gone.

This was a situation that could have ended in tragedy, had the child not remembered that taking merchandise without paying for it is not right, and had she not innocently questioned her would-be kidnapper. To this day, he has not been caught. The child's mother still shops at the same store, but now the little girl walks in front of her, and her daughter, not her shopping list, is her first priority. This woman and her child were fortunate to have survived that potentially tragic encounter, but many others will not be lucky enough to have such a "warning bell." Don't wait for something bad to happen before you begin to understand and act upon the need to keep your child in your direct line of sight and within your grasp at all times.

Though we certainly can't prevent every bump and bruise, either emotional or physical, that a child is likely to experience as a part of growing up, we can learn to provide a loving blanket of awareness that will go a long way toward avoiding those worst possible scenarios. Keeping our children safe is my own highest priority, as it should be, I believe, for all parents.

SHOPPING WITH KIDS: HOW TO KEEP THEM SAFE

1. The most important rule: Never let your child out of your direct line of sight. How close to keep him or her will depend upon the child's age and physical skills (toddlers, obviously, must stay closer than ten-year-olds) and your own (how far and how quickly you can reach). If the child is still small enough to ride in the shopping cart, that's usually the safest place for her. And it should go without saying—never leave the shopping cart unattended!

2. When you're in the store, take note of any strangers or unsavory characters who may interact with your child. Not all strangers are bad guys, but not all bad guys look scary. Most interaction is simply friendly and harmless, but the most harmless-looking person can also be dangerous, so *always* be vigilant of *any* stranger who approaches your child.

3. Make sure your child's fingers don't get caught in the fold-down seat of the cart, and be particularly careful to keep his hands away from moving objects like the belt of the checkout counter. Curious little minds and fingers have a way of wandering, but your child could be badly injured if her hands or fingers get caught in the machinery. I found this out the hard way when I wasn't so little. I was eighteen at the time and working at a parcel company at night while going to college during the day. I was trying to unjam a bunch of packages on the conveyer belt when my left work glove got caught and I broke my pinky and forefinger. If it hadn't been for the fast work of Bill, the shop steward, Tom, the clerk, and John, the mechanic, my fingers would have been completely torn off, probably destroying my chosen career before it had even started. Thanks to them and a good medical team, my hand healed perfectly.

4. When walking to your car, always hold your child's hand with your stronger hand (if you're right-handed, use your right hand), and carry your shopping bag in your weaker hand. (If you are carrying an infant, the same rule should apply: use your stronger arm to carry the child.) Should you have an encounter with a possible assailant or if a vehicle pulls out blindly, you'll be able to protect your child as you maintain your grip on her, and let your bags go. If you have too many packages to hold in one hand, ask the store personnel for help. After all, they are supposed to provide service to their customers.

5. Always put your packages into the car *after* you've safely placed your child in the vehicle. Never let your child stand by the car and out of your sight while you load your packages aboard. Be careful of traffic in busy parking lots. Remember, things like grocery items can be replaced, children can't!

6. Never, under any circumstances, leave your child alone in a vehicle. All too many children get hurt playing in the car while their parent is running a "quick" errand. And, in the worst case, this would be a prime opportunity for a random abduction.

TOM'S TIP

THE ELDERLY TARGET

The elderly are generally targeted for theft of their social security or pension checks, or for whatever cash or valuables they may be carrying on their person. Obviously their age and possible infirmity make them attractive victims, especially for those who have little or no respect for human life.

Last summer I was asked to speak at a senior citizens' home near the town where I grew up, about how elderly people could reduce their risk of becoming crime targets. When I arrived, I was greeted by an audience of more than eighty people who ranged in age from seventy to eighty-five. I started my talk by announcing that if anyone had a question or a story to share, he or she should stop me by raising his hand. As soon as I said that, a stocky, silver-haired lady with a cane put her hand in the air. "Young man," she said, "I would like to tell you what happened to me last week. I was crossing the street to get back home here, when I was trapped by two young hoodlums who pushed me up against the side of the building. First they pulled my cane from me, forcing me to lean against the wall of the building to keep my balance. Then they asked specifically for my social security check, so they probably knew in

SAFETY FOR SENIORS

1. Always travel with at least one other person; larger groups are even better.

2. Take advantage of one another's best senses or resources. For example, if one person sees better, let him be the eyes of the group, and if another hears better, let her be the ears.

3. While traveling, limit your conversation and concentrate on the destination. Since seniors are generally targeted because they are thought to be "easy marks," be attentive and let people know you're watching. Scan your surroundings and always keep your head moving to get the broadest view.

4. Cell phones are now very inexpensive, and having one with pre-programmed emergency numbers—such as your closest relative, the local police, your doctor, and the fire department—is a smart thing to do.

5. Have an emergency contact arrangement in place with a relative or close friend you know you can count on. Pick someone who will deal with the issue quickly and efficiently, and who will not become emotional, thus adding to your problem. Precious seconds and sound decisions save lives.

6. Avoid at all costs areas that are poorly lit or where there are a lot of bushes or trees. Know your surroundings and when in doubt, stay out!

7. If confronted by the bad guy, give him what he wants as quickly as you can. Do not get brazen or bold; in fact, be docile, shaken up, and cooperative, even if that means a little improvisational acting.

TOM'S TIP

advance what day the checks were delivered. I told them my check went directly into my bank account and that I had no money with me at all. But I guess they didn't believe me, because they checked the pockets in my coat, where they found two dollars and twelve cents. One said to the other, 'Man, we can't buy crap with this.' Then the one to my left pushed me down while the other one spit on me. They both laughed and pumped their fists in the air, and then they left me there bleeding from my knee and walked off as if it was nothing to them. I crawled to the front of the house and yelled for help. Two of my friends got me inside and called the police. I know I'm elderly and there's not much that I can do to defend myself short of buying a gun. I just want to know one thing from you, Tom," she said, starting to cry. "Why do people do things like that?"

I walked over to her, and as I got closer I could see the cuts on her leg. I knelt in front of her and took her hand, and said, "It's hard for people who have no respect for themselves to have respect for others. Certain types of individuals believe that life dealt them an unfair hand, and so, to even the score, they take their hatred out on the innocent and the harmless. I'm sorry I can't offer any immediate remedy that will fix your leg or heal your emotional scars."

There was one thing I could promise, however. I asked her how long the lights on the side of the building had been out. A person in the back of the room yelled, "Well over a year." I guaranteed her, and all the other residents, that by the following day the entire perimeter of the building would be well lit. After the talk, I met with the governing body of the home, and the next day all the lights were fixed and the shrubbery was trimmed to allow more visibility in and around the facility.

The best way for the elderly to avoid becoming victims of predators is always to travel at least in pairs, if not in larger groups, because the more people there are, the more difficult it is to disable them. Many elderly people say they're afraid to go out after dark, and that makes a good deal of sense, since potential attackers are less likely to strike when the streets are bright and crowded with potential witnesses.

THE MALE TARGET

One rarely discussed subject is why men become targets. The answer, in many cases, is quite simple. Bad Guests create or take advantage of bad situations. Take, for example, what all too often happens when a bunch of guys go out on the town to have a good time and wind up in an altercation. Why is that such a common scenario? Because alcohol and drugs have different effects on different bodies. When the guys go out for a few drinks, a few can turn into too many, which can lead to some kind of violent altercation.

During college, when I was working in various bars as a security person—a bouncer—I often found myself having to intervene in fights between patrons that had started over nothing. "He looked at me wrong." "He called me a name." "He was looking at my girl." "I don't like the way he looks."

Later on, when I went into protective services and worked at large, elaborate events, I was initially surprised to find myself involved in the same kinds of disturbances. What I learned was that it doesn't matter how old they are or what their income bracket may be; alcohol causes some adults to turn into children. When people get drunk, they get stupid. As I often tell groups, "If you're drinking, you're not thinking."

At a celebrity charity event for which I provided security, one well-known personality was apparently upset to see that the same kind of shirt he was wearing was also being worn by another celebrity. So, to feed his ego, he started telling everyone he spoke to that his shirt had been specially made and the other guy's was a cheap knock-off. Well, news travels fast and soon the other celebrity found out what he was saying and approached him. Within seconds the two were on each other like mortal enemies—all over a shirt.

Both men had been drinking, the one who started the rumor more than the other. And when my team member and I intervened, there was no talking sense to either one of them. Their fight was ego-driven and fueled by testosterone. The person in charge of the event didn't want either of them thrown out, so we separated them gingerly, and, thinking on my feet, I promised each one of them a personal bodyguard for the evening so that they could both enjoy themselves without becoming involved in another altercation. I picked two of my best personnel and assigned them to these gentlemen, and the event continued with no further problems from them or anyone else.

IF YOU'RE DRINKING, YOU'RE NOT THINKING

It's a common fact that guys like to go out for a beer. There's nothing wrong with having a few beers as long as your indulgence doesn't affect your health or that of others around you. According to the National Institute on Alcohol and Alcoholism, alcohol abuse is at its highest in people between the ages of nineteen and twenty-nine, and in fact that statistic is very much in line with what I've encountered professionally. Needless to say, I've dealt with many people whom alcohol or drugs have turned into Bad Guests, and, more often than not, they've been between the ages of twenty-two and thirty. Here are some do's and don'ts for dealing with people under the influence of alcohol.

1. Know when to talk and when to listen. Try to get the person to cooperate, but understand that trying to talk to her as if she were sober usually doesn't work, especially when tempers or emotions are running high. I have always found that the fewer people who try to intervene, the better the result. Too many voices and egos usually just add to the problem.

2. Tell the person you care. If, for example, you don't want the person to drive, tell him you're worried and think it's best that he not drive. Don't keep accusing him of being drunk, because he'll just keep telling you he's not, and then you'll be in for a battle of either wills or fists.

3. Be conscious of the person's every movement. I have found that often someone will appear to be able to walk but will leave the premises and then fall down, causing herself severe injury. If you have a good relationship with her, put your arm around her in a caring gesture and guide her steps. Also, when entering or exiting a vehicle, be sure you remind her to watch her head. I've seen far too many intoxicated people crack their heads open getting into or out of a vehicle.

4. If the person becomes violent, avoid confrontation at all costs. Get someone to help who knows how to help, such as a police officer or a properly trained security person. Do not try to reason with a person who is not thinking clearly. Violent drunks tend to strike out at random and can do serious bodily harm.

5. If someone you know starts destroying property—either your own or anyone else's—call 911 before you even attempt to do anything to stop him. The key here is to be attentive and watch the person's actions to make sure he doesn't grab a gun or a sharp object. I've seen too many innocent people get hurt while trying to stop a drunk from destroying *things* while the one under the influence remains unharmed and very often claims he doesn't even remember doing the deed.

6. Remember that alcohol affects people both mentally and physically, so even if you think you know someone well, she may be an entirely different person after she's been drinking. My best advice is to be caring but always remain cautious.

TOM'S TIP

Males are not free from victimization. Being in the wrong place at the wrong time can cause us to be targeted, as can wearing an expensive piece of jewelry or clothing, or flashing substantial amounts of cash. In fact, most male victims who were in relatively good physical condition have told me that the Bad Guest or Bad Guy had been quick to try to hurt him so that he wouldn't have to worry about becoming involved in a prolonged struggle or the victim's needing to "prove his manhood," particularly in front of his friends or his lady.

In other, more serious cases, those that might be considered a Bad Day, the primary or "alpha" male in the group might be made an example of, just to put fear in the others. This is what often happens in hostage or hijacking situations.

So, even though males are at the bottom of the victim list, they are still on the list, particularly when they become involved in a bad situation or are in the wrong place at the wrong time.

THE TRUTH ABOUT LAW ENFORCEMENT

Most of us hold certain beliefs about what our law-enforcement agencies are supposed to do for us, and, like the woman who was robbed in the garage of the shopping mall, we're quick to cast blame when we or someone we love becomes the victim of a crime. "Where are the cops when you need them?" is likely to be our knee-jerk response. But the fact is that although a "police presence" at large public gatherings or the beat cop are certainly deterrents to crime, the responsibility of the police is not really so much to prevent crime as it is to respond after a crime has been committed.

Captain Mark Prach, a twenty-three-year veteran of law enforcement from New Jersey, and one of the smartest, most honorable law-enforcement officials I've ever met, provided me with some eye-opening information about the number of crimes committed in an average year, and what the police can and can't do about them.

"All of us," he told me, "are in danger, whether we realize it or not. According to the most recent available statistics, there were almost 29 million crimes committed in our country in a single year [1999], more than a quarter of them involving violence against individuals. Altercations occur quickly and unexpectedly. If that were not true, more victims would be able to avoid them. Whether we believe it or not, the fact is that we are vulnerable to having bad things happen to us, and we can't rely solely on others to protect us.

"Analyzing today's society, it's easy to see that we all have to be reasonably responsible for our own safety and well-being. While the police have an overall duty to protect us, the police do not have the resources and cannot be expected to guarantee that no harm will ever come to any particular individual. Various courts have, over the years, determined that, legally, the police—except under very specific and clearly defined circumstances—have no obligation to protect any specific person. Their findings are based on what is known as the 'public duty rule,' which states that the police have a duty to protect the general public but not any particular individual. Without that rule, anyone who was ever a crime victim would be able to sue the police department that was responsible for providing protection in the area where the crime occurred.

"The fact is that there are only so many police officers to go around. In 2001, the U.S. Department of Justice issued a publication titled *Criminal Victimization,* which provided statistics on the amount of time it took the police, on average, to respond to a victim of violence, including rapes, robberies, assaults, and purse snatchings. In just over 70 percent of these cases, it took more than five minutes. In approximately four out of ten cases, it took between eleven minutes and one hour. And, 5 percent of the time, the police responded within a day. Being aware of these figures, it would be both unrealistic and foolhardy for anyone to believe that the police would be there to assist him or her at the moment he or she was becoming the victim of a violent crime. Clearly, therefore, it's up to all of us to do whatever we can to protect ourselves and our families."

CHECKLIST FOR PERSONAL RESPONSIBILITY

✔ *Develop a positive attitude.* The individual whose body language, stance, and expression broadcast self-confidence is less likely to be an attractive target for the criminal seeking a victim. A confident mindset, in combination with a trained body, sends a signal to any potential attacker suggesting that he look elsewhere for his target.

✔ *Develop an effective personal protection plan.* Having a plan in advance will reduce the likelihood that you'll be thrown off guard and act foolishly rather than proactively in the eventuality that you do have to protect yourself.

✔ *Practice protection and evacuation or escape techniques.* "Practice makes perfect" is more than just an old saying. Athletes know that to maintain their skill level they must practice and train on a regular basis. And the same holds true for maintaining the personal-protection skills you'll need should you find yourself or your family confronted by any kind of danger. We're not born with those skills; they must be learned, updated, and practiced.

✔ *Develop your survival instinct.* It's virtually impossible to explain to anyone who hasn't actually been a victim of violence the kind of pressure that kind of situation can produce. While mental and physical training do provide the best tools for ensuring the best outcome, developing a mindset based on a commitment to survive can make all the difference when the pressure is on.

IN SUMMARY

Every one of us must take personal responsibility for doing whatever we can to ensure our personal safety and that of our loved ones. We can't depend on law-enforcement agencies to shoulder that burden for us, and we can't assume that we'll somehow know what to do if we haven't developed and practiced a plan in advance. Like any skill we want or need to acquire, the techniques that will help to ensure our avoidance or survival of a violent confrontation need to be honed through consistent training.

TWO

SAFETY AT HOME

ONE OF MY CLIENTS *was going on vacation. Because we'd discussed it in advance, he was aware of the need to do whatever he could to secure his home from burglars while he and his family were away. So, when the local police in his affluent suburban community informed him that there had been a rash of robberies in the neighborhood, he decided to use his ingenuity.*

He went to the local pet shop and bought three of the largest dog bowls he could find. Just before he and his family left on their trip, he filled the bowls with water and left them in three clearly visible locations outside the house.

When the family returned from their vacation, my client learned that a burglar had been caught trying to break into the house next door to his, and that the thief had actually told the police he'd originally targeted my client's house. He said he'd been keeping an eye on the house and had never seen a dog there, but when he noticed the dog bowls he decided to try the house next door instead.

My client was relieved but also surprised that his little ploy had paid off. He confessed that he'd never thought it would work. But, as he told me afterwards, "I guess the crime profession isn't filled with rocket scientists."

MOST OF US would prefer to believe that even if danger does lurk out there in the world, at least when we're inside our own home we're safe from harm. As a result, too many of us neglect to take the simple precautions that would help to ensure our home safety. When we do that, however, we're putting ourselves and our families at unnecessary risk. Government, law enforcement, and insurance company statistics all rank theft or burglary, fire, and accidental injury, in that order, as the three greatest risks to families. And all of them are most likely to happen in the home.

BURGLARPROOF YOUR HOME

It's never possible to make your home a hundred percent safe from burglars, but, as my client who purchased those dog bowls learned to his relief and delight, sometimes a little forethought can go a long way. And it's equally true that a little neglect can sometimes lead to big regrets. Burglars, as the story above surely indicates, are looking for the path of least resistance, and their choice of targets is most often based upon "golden opportunities" created by our own mistakes or carelessness—a broken window that is not replaced, or an extra key "hidden" in an easily accessible location.

It was just that kind of mistake that caused one of my clients unnecessary distress when he decided it would be tasty fun to start a small vegetable garden in his backyard. There was an ideal spot next to the garage just waiting to be cultivated. He went to the local hardware store and bought himself a selection of tools, then to a nursery where he purchased a variety of starter plants. When he got home, he couldn't wait to begin planting, so he got right to work preparing the soil.

Each day he worked on his garden for a few hours, and when he was done he carefully cleaned his tools and put them away in the garage. One day when his wife was watching him go through this routine, she suggested that since he was using the tools every day, he might as well just wipe them off and leave them by the garden on the side of the garage, which would be a lot easier than dragging them back and forth. Happy to save himself some time and trouble, my client readily agreed.

HOME SAFETY "DON'TS"

To live a safer life and protect what you worked for, look inside and around your own premises and see if you've made one or more of these common mistakes. If you have, correct it *right away*.

1. Don't "hide" an extra key in a commonly accessible location such as under a doormat, on top of a bookcase, behind a shelf, in a hollowed-out fake book, or in an aerosol can.

2. Don't neglect to repair broken locks on windows or doors. What you don't fix today can help a burglar tomorrow.

3. Don't forget to turn on your burglar alarm, and have it updated and/or upgraded regularly.

4. Don't leave the bushes and shrubbery around your house untrimmed, and don't forget to fix outdoor lights.

5. Don't leave your garage or toolshed unlocked. Burglars love for you to make their job easier by providing the tools they need to get into your house.

6. Don't leave your car unlocked, and never leave an extra set of keys to your house in your vehicle. This is a burglar's ultimate dream—the keys to your home!

TOM'S TIP

That Friday the couple went away for the weekend. As bad luck would have it, when they arrived home they discovered that someone had broken into their garage and taken all their lawn equipment as well as anything else of value. The side door had been jimmied open and, next to the door, hidden behind a small bush, was the broken garden tool that had been used to do the job. It was one of the tools my client had bought and left beside the garage. What had seemed like a good idea turned into a bad situation that caused property damage and the loss of valuable merchandise.

We Americans spend millions of dollars every year insuring our possessions—our homes, cars, jewelry, furs—but we don't really think about the fact that when someone breaks into our home, it's not only our possessions but the safety of our family that's at risk.

Law-enforcement statistics indicate that more than 16,000 residences are broken into by burglars every day, and insurance companies report approximately $3 billion lost to theft every year.

Several years ago I stopped in to see my mother, as I did every day when I was in town. On this particular afternoon, a friend whom she hadn't seen for a long time was there for a visit. My mom introduced us and, like other proud mothers, told her friend a little about my work. When she mentioned the word "security," the lady immediately said, "I could have used you when my house was broken into last week." I asked what had happened, and this is the story she told:

It was a rainy night and she decided to go to bed early because she wasn't feeling very well. She was a widow living alone in the same house she and her husband had bought when they first got married. It was about two-thirty in the morning when she heard a noise downstairs. Thinking it must be the wind, she decided to go downstairs and make sure everything was all right. As she walked down the stairs, she saw a flicker of light that she assumed must have been lightning. As she entered the kitchen, she came face to face with a burglar. She screamed, he screamed, and then he ran to the back door, breaking the screen door in his haste to get away. She was gasping for breath, so she leaned against the refrigerator and, once she regained her composure, called the police. When the police arrived, they did a check of the residence with her and found nothing missing. The only damage was the broken screen door. She was lucky in two respects: nothing had been stolen, and, even more important, the burglary hadn't turned into an assault or a murder.

HERE ARE SOME TIPS that will help you to avoid personal injury if someone breaks into your home while you are in the residence:

1. *Stay put.* If you hear a sound and you are alone, lock the door to the room you're in and call 911. Immediately state your full name, your complete address, and why you need help. Leave the phone off the hook so that, if necessary, the call can be traced. If there are children in the house, make the call to 911, then gather the kids into the closest and safest room in the house, and secure it by jamming a chair or another heavy object under the door or the knob as a stopper. The best home-made device is a wedge-shaped piece of wood that you can jam under a tightly closed door. Keep one in each room, hidden and out of the reach of children. Why hide it? First, because you don't want a child to play with it and possibly injure himself or accidentally lock himself in; and, second, because you don't want an intruder to be able to lock you out of the room and possibly prevent you from helping a loved one. (Having recognized the need for a portable, affordable device to secure a door, I worked with my father-in-law, Emil Mueller, a talented and respected tool-and-die maker, to create a unique piece of equipment we call STOP-EM. For futher information, log on to www. tompatire.com/ or www.stop-em.com/.)

2. *Always keep a charged cell phone* in your bedroom at night. There are several reasons for this: An intruder may cut your phone wires. You can take the cell phone with you as you move around. The intruder won't be able to listen in to your conversation by using an extension phone in another room.

3. *Should you not be able to reach your loved ones,* especially a child, think first. Make the call so that you know help is on the way, and then deal with the moment. It's your job to protect those who can't protect themselves, so do whatever it takes to lure the intruder away from the child. The key word here is *stall* so that help has time to arrive. If the intruder becomes violent (though most burglars are nonviolent, you can't know how he'll react if confronted) and you are capable of defending yourself, be prepared to do so. Your desire and motivation are simple— your life and the lives of your loved ones depend on you! I'll provide simple self-defense techniques in chapter six.

4. *Get out.* If the door to exit the residence is nearer than the phone, get out.

5. *If you are confronted* by the burglar, do not make any sudden moves. See what he does and listen to what he says. Remember that no

material possession is worth fighting or losing your life for. Most burglars are in this type of profession because they are nonviolent. That's why they target the homes of people who are away, but sometimes they make a mistake and run into a resident they thought was out or on vacation.

Though burglars don't really want to find you at home, it's impossible to ensure that no one can possibly get in while you're there. As you may recall, even Buckingham Palace proved not to be burglarproof when, several years ago, a young man entered Queen Elizabeth's bedroom while she was sleeping to have a little chat. We can, however, take some simple but effective precautions.

CHECKLIST FOR HOME SECURITY

✔ *Install top-quality, high-security cylinder locks on all exterior doors.* Deadbolts with three-inch screws are excellent for all exterior doors, including sliding doors. And don't neglect to lock the dead bolt when you're inside!

✔ *Be sure your doors are made of metal or solid wood.* Hollow-core wooden doors are for interior use only.

✔ *Reinforce all doorframes.* It would be foolish to install an expensive lock just to have your doorframe splintered by a single well-placed kick.

✔ *Maximize visibility from both inside and outside your home.* In our quest for privacy, we tend to allow trees and shrubs to grow up around our windows. Prune any that obstruct your view from within or might provide a hiding place for a burglar lurking without.

✔ *Keep tools and ladders out of sight, and keep garage or toolshed doors locked.* You don't want to be the one who inadvertently provides the burglar with just the tool he needs to get inside your house.

✔ *Make sure all your entrances are well lit.* Photosensitive lighting units that go on automatically when night falls are very good deterrents to crime, and provide both police and firefighters with greater visibility.

✔ *Install highly sensitive "glass break" detectors.* The tinkle of breaking glass might not be enough to alert you—or your neighbors—to someone entering through a window, but the sound of an alarm going off would surely wake someone, and would scare the intruder into running as well.

✔ *Be sure all hinge pins are inside the house.* There's no point to having a top-quality lock or a metal door if all the burglar has to do is unscrew the hinges on the other side and walk in. Think like a burglar before you install safety devices. If you can bypass them, a professional certainly won't have a problem doing the same.

✔ *Keep an up-to-date inventory of all your valuables, with descriptions, serial numbers, and values.* It's impossible, as I've said, to make your home absolutely burglarproof. In the unfortunate event that a thief does get in, the more information you're able to give the police, the greater will be the chances that your belongings will be recovered. In the stress of the moment, you might well forget something, so it's helpful to have a list. And in any case you'll have to furnish this information to your insurance company when you make a claim.

✔ *Whenever possible, mark each valuable item with a specific code or initial.* Again, this might help the police to identify your stolen property, which could then lead them to the perpetrator of the crime. A friend of mine had all three of his children's bicycles stolen from his parked van and, when he took the kids to a secondhand bike shop to replace them, his daughter saw her stolen two-wheeler among the merchandise. The bike shop owner tried to tell her it was another bike that just looked like hers (after all, if it was her bike, he was clearly in receipt of stolen merchandise), but when she pointed out her name taped to the underside of the seat, he had to admit she had undeniable proof.

BURGLARPROOF YOUR BEHAVIOR

Locks, lights, and alarms are certainly your first line of defense, but your own behavior, both inside and outside your home, can also help to improve your chances of escaping the watchful eye of a potential burglar. You may recall that the woman who was robbed in the parking garage was wearing expensive jewelry and clearly signaling her affluence to anyone who might care to notice. If either your home or your personal style broadcasts your wealth, you just might be attracting the wrong kind of notice. Creating the impression that you have nothing of value will, on the other hand, make you a less attractive target. You don't, after all, want to inadvertently issue an invitation to the wrong kind of "guest."

If you're home alone, try to give the impression that there are more people inside. Light up the entire house, leaving no zones of darkness. Put on the television or radio to bring life into the house. Move from one room to another so that your shadow in the window will indicate activity on different levels and in different rooms. If there is more than one bathroom, use different ones at different times. Random movement is a deterrent to crime because the potential burglar will have to guess where you are at any given moment. If the Bad Guy is watching the house, he already knows you're at home, and limiting your movement will make you an easier mark, so stay active.

An awful lot of us seem to be creatures of habit. If you follow the same routine every day, you just might be making yourself a potential target for an observant burglar. If you're not sure how predictable your own habits are, ask a good friend if he or she knows what you do on a daily basis—what time you go to work; what time you come home; when you walk the dog; when you go to the supermarket, and so on. You might be surprised to discover how predictable you are.

To prove this, I asked each of two women who had been neighbors and best friends for two years to write down the other's daily routine. I sent them to opposite ends of the room and gave them ten minutes to complete the task. When they were done, I asked them to list the names of every person to whom they had mentioned each of these daily events. Finally, I asked each of the women to write down her own daily itinerary. When I compared the two, I discovered that each of these friends knew more than 80 percent of what the

KEEP YOUR HOME SAFE
WHEN YOU'RE NOT THERE TO GUARD IT

Especially when you're away, learn a lesson from my client who went out to buy those dog bowls and make it as difficult as possible for burglars to determine whether or not anyone is at home.

1. Keep the dates of your vacation confidential.

2. Install lights that go on automatically at night. (You can program automatic lighting to go on and off in different rooms at different times on different days. The more random the program, the less likely it is that a criminal staking out the property will be able to determine when—or whether—you're at home.)

3. Before you leave, double-check all doors and windows to be sure they are locked. Set your alarm, if you have one, and notify the alarm company or your local police department of the dates you'll be gone.

4. Store all valuables and firearms in a secure safe that is well hidden from sight.

5. Ask a friend or relative to pick up your mail (or arrange to have it held at the post office).

6. Remember to cancel your newspaper delivery.

7. Ask a trusted neighbor or friend to park his car in your driveway.

8. Have a trusted neighbor, friend, or family member walk your property at different times of the day or night to indicate to anyone who might be watching that your house is being looked after and will not be an easy target.

9. If you do return to find you've been burglarized, *do not touch anything*. Leave the premises and go directly to the nearest phone to inform the police. Remember, there's always a possibility that the burglar is still inside.

TOM'S TIP

other did every day. What is more, each of them had mentioned something about the other's schedule to at least eight other people in the course of a day. Knowing human nature, I'd have to guess that each of those eight then mentioned the same events to eight more. The point is that a Bad Guy or a Bad Guest might gather information about you just by being in the right place at the right time or because he knew someone who was connected to you by up to eight degrees of separation! During World War II, Uncle Sam reminded us that "loose lips sink ships." In my business, I've turned that warning into a motto of my own: "Too much talk allows the robber to steal and walk."

In addition, we tend to talk a lot about our private business—and the business of others—in public places. If you do that—sitting at the counter or in a booth at a restaurant, standing on line at the grocery checkout, or waiting to get into a movie—you might just be giving a sharp-eared thief the information he needs to make you, or someone you know, a target for crime.

CHECKLIST FOR BURGLARPROOFING YOUR BEHAVIOR

✔ *Vary your daily routine, and keep it to yourself or share it only with a trusted loved one.* If a Bad Guy or a Bad Guest is watching and studying you from afar, the key is to keep him guessing by not falling into a pattern of habitual movement.

✔ *Don't display your valuables where they can be seen from outside through a window.* Thieves choose to act for many reasons, but one of the main reasons is that they perceive the opportunity for a quick hit. Something catches the Bad Guy's eye and he shatters a window or pops a door, runs in, and runs out with your valuables. Something you might have saved up for a long time to buy, or something you might truly cherish, will be gone in a few seconds.

✔ *Never let a stranger into your home for any reason—especially one who asks to use your phone.* Bad Guys come in all sizes and shapes; they don't have to appear menacing or scary. Even a service person who is there for a specific reason can turn into a Bad Guest once he's inside your home, and can become a problem rather than fixing yours. A service company should notify you in advance of the time their employee will arrive, and you, as a homeowner, have a right to ask the company for the name and a description of the person they'll be sending, as well as for information about the length of time he's been with the company. Many times, the company will then inform the employee that you've asked these questions so that he'll be on his best behavior.

✔ *If a workman comes to your door, even if you've made a appointment, ask to see his identification.* Identifications come in all shapes and sizes. If you have any doubt about the legitimacy of the one you're being shown, ask the workman for his supervisor's name and direct phone number and call his organization or the local authorities.

✔ *If you receive a "wrong number" call, don't give out any information.* Ask politely what number the caller is trying to reach. If the number is different from yours, instruct the caller to dial again. Should the number be the same as yours, tell the caller that no one by that name lives at the number and hang up at once.

✔ *Don't tempt fate (or thieves) by flashing your cash or bragging in public about what you've got.* Most of the time we keep our money stashed in our purse or rolled up in our pockets. When it comes time to pay for something, we shed light on what we have by reaching for our money without even thinking about who might be standing nearby, or by placing our cash on the counter as we count it. To reduce your chances of becoming a target, be aware of the amount of cash you are carrying. If you carry your cash in your pockets, put bills of smaller denominations, such as ones and fives, in one pocket and larger denominations in another. That way, if you buy something inexpensive, you won't be flashing large amounts of cash unnecessarily. If you keep your money in a wallet, arrange the bills in two sections, with the smaller denominations in the front. In a purse, divide your bills the same way and put them in different compartments. Always have a credit card handy, and always keep it with the smaller bills.

✔ *Keep your private business private by talking less and listening more when you're in public.* We Americans seem to love engaging in conversation with people we don't know. We're just trying to be friendly, but most of us don't think before we talk. We should begin learning to watch what we say, especially when answering questions. Bad Guys get good information simply by listening.

To prove how easy it is to get information from strangers, I'll tell you a true story about something that happened when I traveled to San Diego with Darren Hamilton, a senior member of my training staff who was traveling with me.

We stopped at a pizza shop for lunch and, because it was a beautiful day, decided to eat at an outside table. A few minutes later two young ladies sat down at the table next to ours and engaged us in conversation. Within five minutes one of the girls was showing Darren her driver's license, which is full of personal information, just because he'd said he didn't believe she'd given him her real name.

Within ten minutes the other girl had told me her name and address, what kind of car she drove, that she lived alone, that she had no pets, the layout of her apartment, and what she did for a living.

BEWARE OF SCAM ARTISTS

One of the trainers on my staff recently told me that he'd received a phone call from an individual who claimed to be an AT&T service technician conducting a test on the phone lines. He told my trainer that in order to complete the test he should please touch 9-0-# and then hang up. My trainer was suspicious enough to refuse. As soon as he hung up, he called the phone company and was informed that had he done as he was asked, the person on the other end of the line would have had complete access to his phone line and could have placed a long-distance call to anywhere in the world.

The moral is that if a story sounds fishy to you, don't get sucked into taking the bait.

TOM'S TIP

What this story indicates is that we "good guys" make judgments based on first impressions just as criminals do when they select their victims. In this case the young women had decided we were good guys, with good intentions, and they were right. But before Darren and I left, I gave them some free advice on not being so open to strangers, because strangers who are Bad Guys make it their business to seem like nice, everyday people in order to get potential victims to drop their guard.

PROTECT YOUR PERSONAL INFORMATION

One important aspect of keeping your private business private is protecting your personal information. Most often, when we talk about personal protection, we're thinking about our physical well-being. With recent advances in modern technology, however, it's becoming easier and easier for criminals to acquire enough information about you to steal your actual identity—and use it for their own purposes. In addition, there are still many "low-tech" methods for stealing your identity without ever stealing your wallet. These might include stealing your mail, going through your trash, which generally contains a wealth of discarded personal information, and even stealing information from your employment records.

Finding purchases you never made or services you never used listed on your credit card bill can certainly be disturbing—as it was for my client (a lawyer, no less) who "lost" his wallet only to find thousands of dollars charged to his credit card within just a few days. It may have taken only days to create the damage, but it took him almost two years to undo it and clear his credit record. Even worse, however, the thief may be using your identity when acting illegally or even perpetrating crimes against other people. One of my own employees didn't have a clue that someone else was using his identity until he began to receive tickets from motor vehicle agencies in states he'd never even visited. To prove his innocence he had to hire not only an attorney but also a handwriting expert to prove the signatures on the tickets weren't his.

When I appeared on a television program not long ago, one of my fellow guests was a young woman who'd had her identity stolen by a Bad Guy who'd rung up thousands of dollars in charges on credit cards he'd obtained by using her name. When she checked her credit report and saw all the outstanding debt, she said, she just broke down in tears. It took several years and several lawyers to prove to the irate creditors that the charges weren't hers. On the program she talked about the court cases, all the phone calls to the credit agencies, and the thousands of dollars she'd spent to fight what she called "the process." She said it had been the worst two years of her life, and that even though she was the victim, the "system" had treated her like a criminal.

Taking a few simple precautions can help to ensure that no one's walking around using your good name to do something bad.

CHECKLIST FOR PROTECTING YOUR PERSONAL IDENTITY

✔ Be aware of the people around you whenever you're using your bank card or phone card in a public place. If you have any doubts or feel uncomfortable, go to another ATM or phone booth.

✔ Before writing any of your personal information, such as when you're filling out a form in a public place, glance around to see if anyone is watching.

✔ Avoid writing your personal information while standing in front of a window through which someone might be watching.

✔ Never give out your personal information to a telemarketer, even if you're interested in the service or product. Ask that the information be mailed to you, and ask for a phone number so that you can call back.

✔ Be aware that people who engage in telephone fraud often use a temporary number that's here today and out of service tomorrow. Once you take a number, *don't* call it back. Call the company's headquarters to find out if the number you were given really belongs to one of their employees and whether or not the company is really selling the item or service you were offered.

✔ If you have been a victim of identity theft, call the Federal Trade Commission Theft Hotline toll-free at 1-877-IDTHEFT for immediate professional help.

✔ Never provide any personal information over the Internet except on reputable sites that have documented encryption procedures.

✔ Know that you can identify and locate all your important papers in case you have to determine whether or not they've been stolen or lost.

✔ Immediately report and rectify any bills or tickets you suspect might be illegitimate.

✔ If you know that your wallet or any of your papers have been stolen, immediately notify all credit reporting agencies in your area that an "identity theft alert" should be placed on your file. Once that's been done, no new account can be opened in your name without your personal authorization.

✔ Never throw away any personal paperwork that hasn't been shredded or torn into many pieces. Dispose of the pieces in several different trash baskets. Never dispose of old credit cards, bank cards, or identification cards without first cutting them into small pieces.

✔ If possible, order bank checks printed with your initials rather than your full name, your work phone number rather than your home phone number, and your work address or a post office box rather than your home address. Never, never print a personal identification number such as your social security number on the checks. You can always write it in when necessary.

✔ Maintain an easily accessible list of the toll-free numbers for your credit card companies and banks. Keep a second copy in a safe place at home. The sooner you are able to notify the proper authorities of lost or stolen cards, the sooner they'll be able to take appropriate action.

✔ Call the three national credit-reporting organizations as soon as you can. Direct them to place a fraud alert on both your name and your social security number, and leave a number where you can be reached in case there is any activity on these reports. Once you do that, they'll be alerted whenever anyone tries to check your credit, and the person checking will have to contact you to authorize the new credit. That way, the person who stole your card won't be able to use your good name for bad purposes.

✔ As a safety measure, check your credit report (see below) at least twice a year so that you know what's on it.

✔ Make sure that you file a police report ASAP in the jurisdiction or area where the card was stolen. Thinking clearly and acting diligently can make all the difference when a criminal tries to go on a spending spree that might ruin your credit.

Identity theft can be far more insidious than simply finding that someone's bought a new VCR with your Visa card. Anyone who's had to deal with untangling the knotty problems that can result from a moment's innocent carelessness can attest to the fact that when it comes to safeguarding your own identity, it's definitely better to err on the side of caution.

KEEP THESE NUMBERS HANDY

The three major credit reporting agencies:

➡ Experian (formerly TRW), 1-888-397-3742

➡ Trans Union, 1-800-680-7289

➡ Equifax, 1-800-525-6285

➡ Also, the Social Security Administration Fraud Line, 1-800-269-0271

Call them all!

TOM'S TIP

SAFE SHOPPING

By Phone

1. Know what you are actually getting. If the item you want is no longer available and you're offered something "better," stop and think. Maybe the original item never existed, or maybe the new one isn't really better at all—just more expensive.

2. Don't allow yourself to be pressured. When in doubt, just say *no* and hang up! The "act now" pitch can sometimes save you money, but it can also cause you a lifetime of headaches.

3. Stay away from contests—especially those that require you to make a purchase in order to enter. Many of these have unspoken requirements designed to defraud you in some way. Good companies usually offer good contests.

On the Internet

Letting your fingers do the walking on the keyboard can be an extremely easy and time-saving way to shop, so long as you take the proper precautions. The information superhighway has infinitely expanded the horizons of all kinds of businesses, most of them legitimate, but some that are not. The key to shopping safely on the Internet is mostly a matter of using common sense.

1. Know as much as you can about the business you're dealing with, including how long it's been in operation. Some companies that offer Internet services are very well known, but others, which may in fact be equally reliable, are not. It's up to you to find out who and what they are.

2. Know the company's complaint policy, should they have one. Look for information about how complaints are handled. Not all companies are American-based, so it's important to know how you can get in touch with the right people should you have a complaint.

3. Don't believe hype. Many fantastic deals, giveaways, and even free credit are offered online. As with anything else, if it sounds too good to be true, it probably is.

4. Protect your personal information at all costs. Provide only as much as you need to complete your purchase. If you're not purchasing anything, don't provide any information.

5. Pay the safest way you can. I have found that credit cards are the safest way to pay online. The charges are easy to dispute, and the credit card company will reduce your liability to only fifty dollars if you can prove that the offer was misrepresented. This is a federal law, and the law will protect you.

TOM'S TIP

FIREPROOF YOUR HOME

Making sure that you and your family, your papers and possessions, and your home are safe from thieves and burglars is certainly of paramount importance, but safeguarding your home and your loved ones from the threat of fire can mean the difference between life and death.

Smoke alarms can save more lives than burglar alarms. Most burglars really don't want to hurt you, they just want your stuff. Fire, on the other hand, has no conscience, and it can kill within seconds. Therefore it's absolutely essential that you learn of a fire as quickly as possible so that you have time to evacuate the children, the elderly, and the infirm as well as yourself. A working smoke alarm provides that early-warning system.

A friend once showed me a package of cocktail napkins she'd bought. The napkins were printed with the message "Dinner will be ready when the smoke alarm goes off," a humorous reference to the fact that smoke alarms can be annoying when they think the chicken you're broiling is creating enough smoke to asphyxiate you. But one of the dumbest things any of us can do is to remove the battery from the smoke alarm just because the alarm it provides is sometimes a false one. Avoiding a couple of false alarms can also prevent you from receiving the one that might save your life.

CHECKLIST FOR FIRE SAFETY AT HOME

✔ Make certain your smoke alarms are all in working order.

✔ Make sure there's a working fire extinguisher on every floor of your home, and that it's within reach of everyone, including children who are old enough to use one. Check the pressure gauges every four months.

✔ Pre-program emergency numbers into the speed-dial on all your telephones, and keep a color-coded list taped next to the phones.

✔ Be sure you have a supply of easily accessible flashlights throughout your home, with batteries in working order.

✔ Be certain that all doors are accessible and in working order, especially those in the basement. Many times, when we're in need of extra storage space, we pile items next to or in front of doors we don't generally use. If there's a fire, however, that otherwise unused door might just mean the difference between life and death. Repair doors that are broken or that have become warped or stuck with age or changes in temperature.

✔ Check all wires, cords, and plugs to be sure they're in good condition. Frayed electrical cords and damaged plugs are serious fire hazards.

✔ Turn off and unplug computers and small appliances, such as toasters and coffee makers, whenever you're leaving home for an extended period of time.

✔ Talk with your family about fire prevention and emergency burn treatment.

✔ Visit your local fire station and talk to a firefighter about fire safety in the home. If possible, take your children along with you.

✔ Devise a plan for what to do in case of fire. Go over the plan with your family, especially your children. Some children's bedrooms are not on the same floor as their parents'. Children need to know how to function quickly, without waiting for Mom and Dad to help them.

SMOKE ALARM BASICS

- Make sure the batteries are fresh. Most smoke alarms have a button you can push to test the battery. Newer ones beep when the battery needs to be replaced. I actually change mine once a month just to be safe. I then use the ones I've removed in my son's toys. If a toy stops working, it won't endanger anyone's life.

- My research indicates that most smoke alarms are intended to last 7 to 10 years (that's the alarm itself, *not* the battery). I, however, replace my alarms every couple of years because, like everything else, there are always newer and better models.

- Smoke alarms work on sensors, so be sure to keep them clean, using a hand vacuum or a clean cloth.

- Place one near every bedroom and 10 feet away from every major appliance including the stove.

- If you're placing your alarm on the ceiling, keep it 8 to 12 inches from the nearest wall.

- Avoid placing alarms near heating ducts or air conditioners that might cause them to go off.

- Those who are hearing-impaired should use alarms that have a strobe light rather than a beeper.

TOM'S TIP

One of the main reasons that fire and smoke inhalation are among the leading killers of average families is that people simply don't know what to do when a fire breaks out. Losing your home or your possessions to fire can be devastating. But losing your life or the life of a loved one is always a tragedy. As with everything we do to protect our personal safety, precaution and planning can save lives in the event of a fire.

According to the National Fire Prevention Association, 3,420

Americans lost their lives, and another 16,975 suffered personal injuries as a result of fire in the year 2000. During the same period, property loss to homeowners was estimated at $5.5 billion. Approximately 85 percent of all fire-related deaths occur in our own residences. Fire is a serious subject, as anybody who's ever witnessed one can attest, and knowing what to do in the event of a fire can save your own life as well as the lives of those you love.

I've never forgotten an incident that occurred when I was twelve years old. It was one o'clock on a Saturday morning, and my brothers and I were awakened by an explosion in our neighbor's garage. We jumped up and started for our parents' room, but they were already on their way to get us. My father looked out their bedroom window and saw flames bursting through the roof of the garage. He grabbed a fire extinguisher and ran out the door in nothing but his flannel pajamas, yelling to my mother to call the police and let them know he was on the scene. "Be careful, Phil, I

WHAT YOU SHOULD KNOW ABOUT YOUR FIRE EXTINGUISHER

- Portable fire extinguishers are good for small fires, but they can only do so much and won't really help when a large blaze is raging out of control.

- Some fire extinguishers are water-based and can't be used on grease or electrical fires, where they would do more harm than good. Know what type of extinguisher you have.

- Some fire departments teach people how to operate a fire extinguisher by using the acronym PASS: Pull the pin, Aim, Squeeze, and Sweep the extinguisher from side to side. The biggest mistake you can make when using a fire extinguisher is to aim it directly at the middle of the fire. Sweeping it from side to side helps to control the fire and prevent it from spreading.

TOM'S TIP

CALL THE FIRE DEPARTMENT!

Always—and I do mean *always*—call the fire department, even if you think you can handle it yourself. In fact, I've told my wife to call first and extinguish second.

TOM'S TIP

love you," my mother yelled after him. And, being my father, he called back, "Don't worry, I'll be all right. Just make the call." My brother Tim and I jockeyed for position at the window to get a view of what was happening, but there was too much smoke and mayhem for us to see anything.

Later, my father's partner, Al Nucifora, came over to let my mom know that Dad was okay and to collect his clothes. It seemed that the neighbor's teenage kids had been working on a racing car in the garage. All the doors and windows were closed, and when one of them lit a cigarette, the place went up in flames. My dad had run in with the fire extinguisher and managed to get the boys out. They were rushed to the hospital, where they were treated and released several days later. My father was treated for smoke inhalation and didn't return home until the following morning.

He never once mentioned his heroic act, but he did sit down with my brothers and me to explain what had happened and to make sure we understood how lucky those boys were to be alive. He also stressed how important it was to keep the doors and windows open when working in a garage, and, above all, how dangerous it was to play with matches, or, as these older boys had done, to light one in an unsafe situation.

FIRE SAFETY DO'S AND DON'TS

- Don't leave the stove unattended while cooking. Even if you have to leave the room to attend to other chores, be sure to check on it at least every 5 minutes.

- *Never* leave the kitchen at all when you are deep-fat frying.

- *Never* smoke in bed or on the sofa, especially if you've been drinking or have taken sleep medication. Better yet, don't smoke at all.

- If you use portable space heaters, keep them at least 6 feet away from any fabric-covered furniture, clothing, or anything else that might catch fire.

- Be very careful when you're using candles. Make sure all candles are extinguished before you leave the house or go to bed. Keep them away from flammable items such as paper napkins, decorations, or draperies. Never put live candles on your Christmas tree. Make sure all candles are in sturdy, nonflammable holders that will catch the wax as it drips. Keep them out of reach of children, and never leave a child unattended in a room where a candle is burning.

- Never leave the house or go to bed when there's a fire burning in the fireplace, even if you think it will "burn itself out."

- Christmastime can be dangerous. Make sure you always keep water in the stand for your tree, and don't keep a tree in the house after it's dried out. As a general rule of thumb, it would be wise to dispose of your tree on January 1.

- Never store fireworks in the house. Keep them far away from flammable solvents, and always be sure they're in a fireproof box or container and out of the reach of children.

- If you burn leaves or garbage (this is illegal in many communities), always make sure it's contained in a cement, dirt, or rock-lined pit that's deep enough to prevent the material from blowing away.

TOM'S TIP

CHECKLIST FOR FIRE EMERGENCIES

✔ Remain calm. Take a moment to gather your thoughts. If you act in panic, you're more likely either to leave yourself trapped or to forget a loved one inside.

✔ Have a system in place for locating your loved ones, or prearrange a meeting place just in case you lose track of one another. In an emergency, your emotions can prevent you from thinking clearly. Having a plan in place will help you to think rationally even under stress.

✔ Have a preset plan and a backup plan. Make sure *all* family members are familiar with both plans, and run through the entire drill at least once a month. Practice your evacuation plans under various conditions, such as in darkness, in different seasons, and in various types of weather.

✔ When evacuating, don't waste time dressing. Put on some footwear if it's readily available, forget the valuables, and get out of the house.

✔ If smoke has begun to fill the residence, stay low to the ground during your evacuation.

✔ When approaching closed doors, feel the door before you open it. If it's hot, try another route, such as through a window. If you have no other option, kick the door open or wrap something—like a shirt or a jacket—around your hand to open it.

✔ When moving in a group, the oldest or most experienced person should go first, followed by the children, with the second-most experienced person bringing up the rear.

✔ Agree in advance on a safe and secure designated location outside the residence where everyone can meet for a head count.

✔ If your clothes catch fire, STOP, DROP, and ROLL.

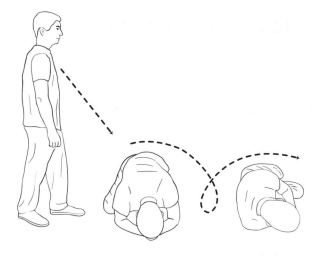

Stop, Drop, and Roll

FIRE DRILLS SAVE LIVES

It's tempting, when you're working at your desk, to "pass" on attending the fire drills most places of business hold periodically. Don't do that! If there really is a fire, you may not have time to think about where the nearest exit is, or what you're supposed to do. Fire drills are intended to educate you before there's an emergency so that you'll be able to act quickly and properly when there is one.

A friend once told me what happened when there was a fire in the high-rise building where she worked. She and her co-workers had become so used to the fire alarms going off "by mistake" that they stopped paying attention to them entirely. Then one day there really was a fire, and the only way she knew it was not a false alarm was when she saw people in the building across the street holding up a large sign that said YOUR BUILDING IS ON FIRE! Luckily, she and everyone else got out unharmed, but not paying attention to the alarm could have resulted in tragedy.

TOM'S TIP

GENERAL HAZARDS IN THE HOME

According to the National Safety Council, approximately 29,500 fatalities and 7,100,000 disabling injuries occurred in the home in the year 2000. In the home, a fatal injury occurs every eighteen minutes and a disabling injury every four seconds. Medical statistics indicate that the most frequent causes of home fatalities are poisons (solid and liquid), accidental falls, fires and burns, and suffocation caused by ingested objects, food or otherwise. The number-one cause is poisoning. Here are some tips for making your residence as hazard-free as possible:

CHECKLIST FOR GENERAL HOME SAFETY

✔ *Chemicals.* Keep any substances that contain poisons in a secure location with childproof latches. Make sure the storage area is sealed, and if ventilation is required, be sure it is outside so the toxic materials do not filter into your living space.

✔ *Slips and falls.* Make sure you have sturdy handrails by all stairwells, and that they are the right height—36 inches is what I recommend to my clients. Use safety gates to prevent children from gaining access to dangerous areas or those in need of repair. Use nonslip mats under loose rugs and in showers or bathtubs.

✔ *Windows.* Install window guards to prevent children from falling out, and keep your windows securely locked. Keep the cords for window blinds or draperies, which can be strangulation hazards, out of the reach of children.

✔ *Electricity.* Make sure the cords on all appliances are in good repair and that all accessible outlets have safety locks to prevent children from poking a toy, a finger, or some other object into them. For greatest safety, check outlets and the cords on your appliances once a week.

THREE

STAYING SAFE OUTSIDE THE HOME

A FAMILY OF FOUR—*a husband, his wife, and their two small children—were attending an amateur softball game in their small town. The parents were chatting and not really paying much attention to what was going on in the field when a batter was thrown out at first and became enraged by the umpire's call. As he walked back to the dugout, he snatched up his discarded aluminum bat and hurled it over the fence and into the stands. The bat struck the husband on the shoulder and bounced off to hit his wife in the head, knocking her unconscious and causing her to fall over on top of her children. The husband, meanwhile, became so furious that he jumped the fence and took off after the batter, oblivious of the injuries his family had suffered. The batter in turn raced to his car and took off, and only then did the husband return to the stands to find his wife bleeding from the head and his children understandably hysterical.*

HAD THE PARENTS in that true story been more vigilant in the first place, they could have ducked the flying bat and provided a shield for their children; had the husband gotten his priorities straight, he'd have attended to his family before taking off on a futile chase; and had these people been familiar with what I call Family Protection Training, they could have avoided the whole traumatic and potentially tragic situation. Like too many of us, however, that father was so focused on one thing—in this case, revenge on the batter—that he was completely unaware of his surroundings and his loved ones.

TRAINING TOGETHER TO PROTECT YOURSELF AND YOUR FAMILY

Most of us simply don't want to consider the fact that every time we leave home with our families, we're putting ourselves at risk for some kind of harm, either accidental or intentional. And I certainly wouldn't want to suggest that anyone should be afraid to go out in public. As a personal protection expert, however, it's my job to make sure my clients—who are often high-profile people—are kept safe in public places, and I know that preparation is the key not only to emerging unharmed from a dangerous situation, but also to maximizing your sense of confidence so that you won't be fearful and inadvertently make yourself a victim.

Since most people wouldn't want to travel around with a team of bodyguards even if they could afford to, I advise everyone to adopt a Training for Life mentality by following the simple steps I've developed for my unique system of Family Protection Training, and to make these precautions a part of their normal, everyday routine. (Although I call this system Family Protection Training, many of these techniques, such as "Training Your Senses," will be valuable for almost everyone, including singles and seniors, so please take the time at least to read it through to see which sections will benefit you.)

It Takes Teamwork

On any team, each player must understand and become adept at the role he or she has been assigned. This is as true in the game of life as it is in baseball or football. The more members of the family—or team—are trained, the more secure the entire family will be.

Family members can function as a cohesive unit to provide mutual protection only if each person on the team accepts his or her role and performs it properly. To do that takes practice, just as it takes practice to hit, catch, or throw a ball with accuracy.

In a typical family situation, the team will consist of two adult parents or guardians and one or more children. One adult is assigned the role that I call Security. The second adult plays the role of the Blanket.

Security's job is to concentrate on the family's destination and surroundings. He or she is the one who will be responsible for performing distraction techniques, if necessary, and for acting as the family's protector. The role of Security is to do exactly what the word says, to "secure" the environment and make it safe for his or her loved ones.

The Blanket's job is to keep the children within direct eye contact and close enough to the adults to avoid involvement with strangers or potentially dangerous situations. His or her responsibility is to provide a comfort zone—physical, mental, or emotional, as necessary—for the children in whatever situation might arise. This is also the person who will be responsible for "cover and evacuation," if that should become necessary.

Security and the Blanket working in combination create a "security blanket" or "comfort zone" for the entire family wherever they may be. Note their unique roles, described below. We'll return to these concepts later in this chapter.

Security

- concentrates on destination and surroundings
- constantly surveys and "reads" the environment
- is responsible for distraction maneuvers
- acts as the family's protector
- makes his (or her) presence known so that anyone who might be watching will know he is paying attention to his environment

The Blanket

- keeps children at a safe distance, within direct eye contact
- is responsible for cover and evacuation maneuvers
- creates a physical and emotional "comfort zone" between children and danger
- distracts the child by whatever means possible from focusing on an upsetting situation
- always puts the child's safety first and foremost

Protecting the Gift

In Family Protection Training, we call children the "Gift." Children are a precious gift to us, and our job is to keep them safe. To do this, we must teach them how far from their parents or guardians they're allowed to wander, but we must also protect them from fear of potential dangers. Their role is to stay close enough for safety so that they can enjoy being children and focus on the fun of discovery without putting themselves in harm's way. As adults, however, we need to remember that children's movements are, more often than not, unpredictable, so keeping them within reach is a chore in itself unless we train them at an early age to develop good, safe habits.

When it comes to keeping children close enough for comfort and protection, the distance will vary with the situation. In a crowded area such as an amusement park or a shopping mall, where there is a lot of activity, I believe it should be less than three feet. In an open area such as a park or field, on the other hand, where there are just a few people scattered about, it might be as far as twelve feet.

When we're in a relaxed and supposedly "safe" environment, it's easy to assume our children are safe and to "let them out of our sight" while we go about our business, but that kind of carelessness can lead to needless panic, as I discovered a few years ago when I was picnicking in a local park with a few other families.

We were all having a good time when suddenly one of my friends realized he couldn't find his seven-year-old daughter. Immediately, everyone scattered to look for the missing child, but there wasn't any plan in place, and after twenty minutes she still hadn't been found. At that point I took over and assigned two-person teams to search specific areas while one adult went to call the police. Luckily, just as law enforcement arrived, the little girl was discovered asleep in the backseat of her parents' SUV, which had been left unlocked. Apparently she'd just been worn out from the day's activities and decided to take a nap. The whole frightening situation would have been avoided if the child had been kept in sight, and the ensuing panic could have been averted if there had been a search plan in place.

Having a Plan of Action

In the realm of family protection, most situations must be evaluated on the spur of the moment and adjusted as necessary. To do that effectively, it's important to have a predetermined and practiced but flexible plan of action in place. You'll need to develop both visual and verbal cues that are easy to remember but "coded" so that no one but your family will be able to "read" them.

Children are really very smart and actually pick up on things even faster than adults. I found this out one day when I was shopping at a mall and ran into someone I'd previously had to remove from a black-tie event where I was working security because of his conduct. The minute he saw me, he decided to voice his opinion—in an increasingly louder voice—of what I'd done. Because I was with my son, who was five years old at the time, I made it a point to cover his eyes as I started to walk away. (Young children are very impressionable. I shielded my son's eyes in this situation because I didn't want to expose him to an increasingly frightening stranger. Later in this chapter I'll offer further explanation and provide more specific information about how to protect children both physically and emotionally.) The man, however, wouldn't let it go and began to follow me to my car. At this point I realized that silence was no longer the appropriate response, so I made it clear that I was with my son, and that if I felt his life were in any way threatened, I'd do whatever was necessary to protect him.

I stopped walking and moved my son behind me. The other man and I stared at each other for about seven seconds, and then, without another word, he left. Following him with my eyes, I picked my little boy up and walked to the car. He was so silent that I got into the backseat with him and asked if he was all right. That's when I learned something. "Dad, was that a bad man?" he asked. I said, "Well, he was a bad man for just a little while." Tommy then said, "I knew he was bad because you made a bad face and you only do that when you see bad people."

What my son was telling me was that he'd read my facial expression, and that was one thing I'd never talked to him about. So, when we got home, my wife and son and I all sat down in the comfort of our own home and talked about the "bad face."

When I talk with my son about the not-so-pleasant aspects of life, I always sit him down in a comfortable environment with my wife, Doris, at his side. She is his natural comfort blanket and very intuitive about helping to explain difficult and delicate issues. I make sure he is attentive to what I'm saying and, most of all, I do it in a non-scary environment. I am certainly not a child psychologist, but here are a few tips I've picked up through life experience that might make it easier for you to talk with your child about delicate subjects.

1. Make sure you pick a place within your child's comfort zone, and that you have his undivided attention.

2. Children understand more than we give them credit for, so you really need to explain the entire situation. If you leave something out or try to downplay it, a child will notice.

3. Do not be afraid to say you made a mistake or that you used "bad language." Sometimes our temper gets the better of us and we need to acknowledge that these things do happen.

4. If you do something inappropriate, make sure you say "I'm sorry." We tell our kids to do that, so we ought to lead by example.

5. Ask your child questions to find out what he's thinking. I taught my son at an early age that asking questions isn't prying, it's protecting.

6. When you've said what you have to, change gears. I do this with my son by telling him a story. The story should be funny and heart-warming, and have a moral. There's nothing better for clearing the mind (both conscious and subconscious) than laughter.

7. After your child goes to bed, check on him periodically to make sure he's sleeping soundly. Usually a child will talk in his sleep or whimper if something has scared him or he has something on his mind.

No matter how hard-nosed or impervious to emotion I have to be in my business, I know that I have to leave that side of my personality behind once I enter the door to spend time with my family. I was reminded of how true this was, not only for me but for all of us, when my family was invited to the home of one of my clients. John Vaughan is a tough businessman and a consummate professional, and when he's making a deal he thinks with his head, not with his heart. I'd never seen him in a family environment, so I wasn't quite sure what to expect, but from the minute we arrived, he, his wife, and their four children all made us all feel like part of their family. He was as gentle and loving with them as he was tough and professional in business, and seeing him and his family together reinforced for me how important it is to check business at the door and create a warm and supportive environment for those you love.

Communicating with Visual Cues

Direct line-of-sight cues are always the most effective in a threatening situation. If possible, look directly into the eyes of your spouse

VISUAL CUES YOU CAN USE

Of course, you can make up your own personal signals in consultation with your partner. Just make sure they are easy to remember, simple to execute, and straight to the point. Here are a few that I've found work very well.

- Look at your partner and touch the outside corner of your eye. Touching your right eye with your index finger would mean that he or she should look to her right; touching the left would mean look to the left.

- Touch your back pocket or hip with the same finger to signal "Look behind you." Again, left or right would signal the proper direction.

- Hold up your index finger and twirl it in a circle to signal "Take a good look around you."

- Put your hand up, palm out, in the "stop" position to signal "Stop in your tracks and don't move or turn around to look."

TOM'S TIP

(or other co-guardian) while making your face expressionless. This facial cue will signal your partner that you believe something is seriously wrong, regardless of which one of you is Security or Blanket. In my experience, direct eye contact and changing your expression are the keys to signaling danger. You can also use these techniques very effectively with even very small children. To prove this, ask your child to laugh and laugh along with him. Then make your expression very serious and watch how quickly the child's attitude and expression change, too.

Although hand signals are often less effective than direct eye contact, they are the next best choice if eye contact isn't possible. The signals should be performed close to your body so that they won't be obvious to anyone except those for whom they're intended. Keep the number of signals to a minimum, and make sure they are simple and easy to remember. Practice them in advance, and make sure each member of your family understands what each cue is intended to signify, such as "Stop," "Come here," or "Stay close to your mother [or father]."

Communicating with Verbal Cues

There may be times when it's not possible to use either direct-line-of-sight cues or hand signals, and in such cases verbal cues are your next best option. The reason they're less desirable than visual cues is that the person posing the threat will also be able to hear them, and we can't know in advance if his response will be to run from the situation or to escalate the danger. To diminish the possibility of that happening, you should "encode" your predetermined verbal cues so that the bad guy is less likely to recognize your signal.

The best kind of verbal cue to use with your child would be a word you know he'll react to instantly. A friend of mine, for example, calls his son Mikey, but their predetermined cue to use when there's trouble is for him to call the boy Michael. They arrived at that signal when, after going through Family Protection Training, my friend sat down with the seven-year-old and asked him how he knew when his daddy was being serious. "Well," the boy said, "when you and I are playing and having fun, you call me Mikey, and that makes me feel good inside. But if I don't listen, you call me Michael, and that's how I know you aren't playing anymore." Having your child come up with the signal is a good idea because only he or she really knows what's going to draw his attention. Once the word has been agreed upon, be sure you use it only when necessary. Don't take advantage of it just to discipline the child. If you do that, when there really is something dangerous going on, your child might just assume he's done something "bad" and choose to ignore you instead of responding.

A good verbal cue to use with your spouse would be the name of a friend or relative who is either deceased or lives far away. Let's assume, for example, that your grandmother had passed away and her name was Susan. You and your family are walking in a park

VERBAL CUES YOU CAN USE

The key to a good verbal cue is that it should *not* be a word or a reference to something that would come up in the normal course of your conversation. The fact that it's unusual will immediately alert your partner to the danger you've spotted.

- If you're a dog lover but don't like cats, use a word that's related to cats or to some other animal you *don't* like.
- Use the name of a restaurant where you had a memorably *bad* meal.
- Mention a sport you neither play nor watch.
- Use an ice cream flavor you would never order.
- Say the title of a movie you hated.

TOM'S TIP

and you notice a group of rambunctious teenagers heading your way. Instead of alerting the entire family and possibly frightening the children, you might say to your spouse, "Look behind you. I think I see your grandmother Susan." Because you've agreed on the cue in advance and your spouse knows that Grandma has not been around for a while, she or he will be immediately alerted to the potential danger and primed to perform his or her assigned role in your protection plan.

The times when verbal cues will serve you best—even better than visual ones—are in those situations where you determine things are likely to go bad really quickly. Because the hand really is faster than the eye, it will take your partner or spouse a precious second or two to process and respond to a visual cue. Not only do we pick up verbal cues through a broader spectrum than visual cues because our vision is more narrowly focused than our hearing, but it has also been my experience that preplanned verbal cues bypass the recognition/response process and embed in the memory more quickly than visual signals, which cuts down the response time.

Generally speaking, we are a reactive society, and the criminal element knows that. Because, in most circumstances, the criminal is acting and you are reacting, he will normally have a couple of seconds in which to create fear and mayhem in your body and mind. He loses that advantage if you have a plan in place and are therefore able to act rather than react. You have then, in effect, caught him by surprise and forced him to reexamine the situation. If you present yourself as a victim who is likely to become a predator, he will most likely decide to leave you alone and find another victim who is weaker and less well prepared.

CHECKLIST FOR FAMILY PROTECTION TRAINING

✔ When teaching and practicing the Family Protection techniques I've outlined in the preceding pages, be sure that the atmosphere is disciplined without being frightening—particularly to the children. That doesn't mean, however, that you should present it as a game. Your children should understand that this is serious business.

✔ At least once a week, no matter how busy your schedules, everyone in the family should make time to gather together to discuss what is going on in the world, in your particular area, and in the lives of each member of your family. Spotlight a specific imaginary scenario, talk about it, and act out the various potential outcomes. Having done that, you can demonstrate how Family Protection techniques can be used to change a bad outcome into a safe one.

✔ Be sure your children understand that it is your love for them that's causing you to emphasize the serious need for this kind of training. Use real-world examples from television and newspaper reports to explain why it's so necessary. Try to keep the atmosphere relaxed, and don't force your children to concentrate too long. About fifteen to twenty minutes is the longest these sessions should last. After that, their attention will wander and they'll become bored and resentful. My training theory is that "less is better." Less time with just enough knowledge will go a long way.

✔ When you discuss the reasons for engaging in Family Protection Training with your family, be sure to concentrate on the positive rather than the negative situations that might necessitate your using these techniques. You don't want to talk about the potential dangers posed by strangers, but about potentially dangerous situations. When you're acting out a situation, always focus on a positive outcome. What you don't want to say is, "If you don't do this right, the bad guy will hurt you." Unless you're taught always to believe in your actions and never—I do mean *never*—give up, your mind will fall prey to negative thoughts more quickly than it will assimilate positive ones. What you want to teach your family is that if they truly believe in their ability to act, and if that belief is backed by an arsenal of proven techniques, they will be able to keep themselves safe. And always end your training sessions on a happy and positive note. If the session ends with an argument or disagreement, everything you might have accomplished will be washed away by the overriding negativity.

✔ Educate your family by practicing safety and awareness drills. We've all read about safety drills and what families should do in case of a problem in the home. We might even talk about what to do over dinner, but few of us ever practice what we preach. You can make your practice sessions fun by, for example, telling your family that you're going to take them out for ice cream, but that they have to leave the house in fire-drill formation. I do an awareness drill with my family when we're sitting in a restaurant. I ask questions like "Where is the closest exit?" "How many entrances and exits do you see?" Those questions help to raise their awareness while keeping the atmosphere pleasant and relaxed. I have found in my studies that people— especially kids—learn more when they're not under pressure. Reward your family with hugs and kisses. They need to understand that this kind of training is done out of love, and that it isn't boot camp.

✔ Make sure you educate each member of your family on a level he or she can understand. Children, for example, might say they understand what you mean just to end the discussion because, in reality, they're overwhelmed or confused. Make sure they understand that they should never be afraid to come to you with any question or problem they might have.

KEEP IT AGE-APPROPRIATE

Most children younger than ten won't grasp or remember an abstract concept unless you can relate it to something in their everyday experience. For little kids that's often a favorite television show or video. Children love to mimic their favorite characters. So if, for example (depending on your child's preferences), you were to explain how the character Steve from *Blue's Clues* would do the task you're teaching your child, it would be easier for him to understand what you're asking him to do, and more fun for him to do it.

Also, try to keep it simple. Remember that your primary goal is to teach the child to go to the Blanket when you give a particular signal. Try to make practicing short and sweet.

Teenagers will appreciate being treated more like adults and made to feel responsible. Explain that this training is not only for them but to help keep the entire family safe. Show them you trust them by teaching them how to scan the environment. Giving teenagers positive reassurance, helping them to build confidence and trust in themselves, will build character they can take with them into their adult lives when they may take on the role of parent or guardian.

TOM'S TIP

✔ When teaching your children about safety, always lead by example. Many people, for instance, insist that their children wear a helmet when riding their bikes, but then ride along not wearing one themselves. The child then "learns" that when he gets older, he too will be able to buck the system—and might even try it when his parent isn't looking and risk serious injury. Children need to understand that wearing a helmet is a law, not a choice.

TRAINING YOUR SENSES

The success of your Family Protection Training will depend on how alert you are to potential dangers, which means that it's important to train your three main senses—sight, hearing, and smell—to provide you with the best, most accurate information.

Sight

Our eyes provide us with visual information that is sent to the brain and causes us to respond. On the most basic level, that's why we're taught to "look both ways" before stepping off the sidewalk and crossing the street. The problem is that our eyes can also fool us, playing tricks with our mind and causing us to panic unnecessarily. As an example of how that might work, consider this scenario: You're going to pick up your child at school. You do this every day, and every day you enter through the side door. Today, however, the side entrance is being repaired, so you have to enter through the front door. You've been to the school literally hundreds of times, but today everything seems different. Your eyes have gotten used to following a particular pattern, and suddenly that pattern has changed. For the next few minutes you walk around aimlessly. You're still confused, and now you're actually beginning to get nervous. This happens because your eyes are sending an unfamiliar picture to your brain. Even though your mind thinks it's in familiar territory, your visual image of the school has been altered. Finally, you ask someone who points to the classroom around the corner.

If, after walking through the front door, you'd stopped to figure out where the side entrance was and where your child's classroom would be, your eyes would have focused more directly on getting you to your destination. Instead, however, you chose to "wing it," which, in many cases, is not the best choice.

Our eyes are naturally trained to scan from left to right. That's how people in most Western countries are taught to read, which means it's how we are taught to process information. It's a preset motion that's instilled in us from the moment we begin to read. Trying to view our surroundings from right to left is as difficult as trying to read from right to left and comprehend what we've read.

To test the truth of this, go to a location where there's a lot of activity and scan your surroundings from right to left. Then turn away and write down as much information as you can remember. Wait a couple of minutes and scan the same scene from left to right. Turn around and repeat the process of writing down what you saw. I guarantee that your memory will have improved dramatically.

Knowing how to use your naturally trained vision to register and recall even apparently insignificant details can make an enormous difference in a number of situations. Accurate visual cues will most often be your first indication of impending danger. Being confident about the "truth" of what you see will allow you to act on those cues without hesitating or trying to second-guess yourself, and very often a quick reaction makes the difference between avoiding or being caught up in a potentially life-threatening situation.

In addition, the first impression you make on a potential attacker can mean the difference between his choosing to target you or looking for another victim. When you're scanning with confidence, your eyes will be piercing and authoritative, reflecting the belief you have in your body and mind. Without proper training, you'll blink more frequently and look away, hoping to avoid the potential problem. Many victims with whom I've spoken had one thing in common: they stated that they could not accurately describe their attacker because they'd been afraid to look at him.

A former client of mine once went to a football game at a major stadium. Once she was inside, she realized she'd left her cell phone in the car. Since her husband didn't want to miss the kickoff, she decided to go back and retrieve it herself. As she hurriedly moved through the parking lot toward her car, she passed a group of men who were still tailgating and who seemed to be rather intoxicated. They made a few rude remarks, but when the woman continued walking without even giving them a glance, one of the men became so irate that he threw a half-full beer bottle at her. Luckily he missed his target, but he did shatter the front window of her car.

The woman then ran to the nearest security officer, who called the police. When the police arrived, they and the security guard returned with the woman to her car. The men were still there partying, but when the police asked the woman which one of them had thrown the bottle, she couldn't tell them. Nor could she tell them who had made the rude comments. The police then calmly looked at her and said, "Miss, in the future you should pay more attention to your surroundings and less attention to your cell phone."

In another situation, a mother's ability to recall details brought about a much happier conclusion when her nine-year-old daughter was abducted while playing outside her house. As soon as the little girl's mother realized she was missing, she called the police, who arrived within minutes. She was able to give them a complete description of what her child was wearing, from her yellow beret to the gold chain around her neck, to the kind of shoes she was wearing.

A neighbor who had noticed the police car in the woman's driveway came over to see what was wrong and rounded up others in the neighborhood to begin a search. The police officer on the scene wisely suggested that the searchers look for little things like the beret, pieces of clothing, or the small gold chain the child was wearing. As luck would have it, one of the neighbors found the yellow beret just two blocks away, outside a house. As the police were approaching the house, they saw a car pulling out of the driveway. They blocked the exit with their vehicle and got out to speak to the driver. Looking in the window, one officer thought it odd that the female passenger was in the backseat with a blanket balled up next to her. He asked both the driver and the passenger to step out of the car, and that's when the driver made a run for it. One police officer chased the man on foot as the other detained the female and searched the car. Rolled up inside the blanket, bound and gagged, was the missing girl. She'd been stripped of her clothing and wrapped in an old flannel nightshirt, but she was thankfully neither hurt nor sexually abused. The key to her successful recovery was her mother's attention to detail and her ability to provide an accurate description to the searchers.

As I was developing my theory of scanning, I experimented with different ways of "looking" before I determined that scanning from left to right definitely allowed me to retain the most accurate picture of what I'd seen. Then, when I worked with making eye contact during a direct confrontation, I found that staring into someone's eyes to let him know you mean business takes a great deal of discipline and concentration, and that it didn't work for everyone. Rather, I determined that looking *through* someone—glancing at the person's upper chest and over either his left or right shoulder at a forty-five-degree angle—gives you a look of authority and confidence as well as a full view of the person's body, allowing you to see most of his actions at all times. I believe that looking up gives you a better view because your eyes are open wider than when you look down.

Scanning

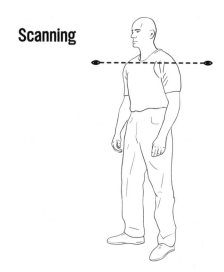

So, whether you're looking at your surroundings or at a particular person, don't stare. Staring tires the eyes, which leads to unclear or fuzzy sight. Glancing, on the other hand, is a more relaxed way of looking, which provides a clearer picture in a shorter length of time. I've found that by teaching people to glance rather than stare at their surroundings, I've gotten better results and my students have been more comfortable with what they were doing. Simply being more relaxed allowed them to gather and process more accurate information.

You can practice glancing by looking through a window into a shop or a room. You'll find that looking slightly up and at an angle rather than straight ahead at eye level will give you the best view.

Should you, however, find yourself in a situation where you want another person to see that you're aware of what's going on around you, you'll need to replace your glance with a glare of caution that will let the person you're "sizing up" know you've taken a total, methodical look at him and the immediate surroundings. By doing this, you are also telling your brain to store the information. Again, your scan should move from left to right and should be slow but steady. Should you need to concentrate on a particular angle, stop, process, and move on. Think of your eyes as a moving video camera that's storing information in your brain instead of on film.

There may, however, come a time when a blank stare aimed directly at a potential predator can be a lifesaver. It worked to my advantage when, a couple of years ago, my wife and I took a ride into New York City to see the Christmas tree at Rockefeller Center. As is typical during the Christmas season, there was a long line of cars waiting to enter the Lincoln Tunnel. We were crawling toward the tollbooths when a car stalled in front of us, making it necessary for me to move into another lane. The driver to my left politely motioned for me to move in front of him, but just as I was maneuvering to do that, the driver to my right tried to cut me off, causing all traffic to come to a complete halt as he and I stared each other down. That driver then decided to get out of his car and walk over to my car. When he got to my window, which was rolled up because it was cold, he looked into my car and starting yelling profanities and verbal threats while I just stared into his eyes with a completely blank expression. Within fifteen to twenty seconds he stopped shouting and his entire demeanor changed. He looked at me and said, "You must be nuts. You're not worth my time." Then he turned abruptly and got back into his car, even allowing me to pull in front of him. During the entire altercation, I had not uttered a single word. My wife always jokes about my nutty-looking stare, but in this instance that stare allowed both of us to remain safely inside our car and prevented a potentially volatile situation from escalating even further.

CHECKLIST FOR ACCURATE VIEWING

✔ Always scan from left to right.

✔ Look through objects rather than directly at them.

✔ When scanning your surroundings, use a glance rather than a stare.

✔ Constantly change your viewing angle in order to get an all-around view of your surroundings.

✔ Use a slow-moving glare to let a potential Bad Guy know you're aware of what he's doing.

✔ When using your eyes to deter a Bad Guy or Bad Guest, stare directly into his eyes with a blank expression on your face.

✔ When moving from the light into darkness, close one eye. This will make it easier for your eyes to adjust to the dark.

✔ Never stare directly at a bright light. Doing that will only blind you. Always look down and away from the source of light.

✔ Whenever possible, use reflections from windows or mirrors to give you a better view of whoever or whatever might be lurking behind you.

Hearing

Like sight, hearing can also play tricks on the mind. One of the most important rules for maximizing the accuracy of our hearing is to control our breathing. As I discussed in the opening chapter, when we perceive any kind of danger, our nervous system sends chemical signals to the brain that affect us physically. One of those physical symptoms is an increase in the pace of our breathing. If you've ever been in a dangerous situation, or even if you momentarily thought you were, you'll probably remember that your heart began to pound so loudly that it was virtually the only thing you could hear. This can also happen if you're sitting quietly relaxed and suddenly hear a loud noise. I call it the "startle effect." If you can train yourself to take deep, slow breaths, your heartbeat will return to normal and your hearing will clear. The more prepared you are, the more you practice Family Protection Training, the less likely you'll be to panic and literally lose control of your senses.

A second cardinal rule for optimizing your hearing is to put yourself at the same height as the sound you are trying to hear. If, for example, you're looking for a lost child who might be calling for you, standing upright, at adult level, will put you far above the trajectory of his voice. And the same would, of course, hold true if you want the child to hear you. Standing upright and screaming into the air so that your voice bounces off or is absorbed by trees, walls, or buildings, at a height way above your child's level, is almost sure to mean that the sound will be lost to him or her.

To be sure that you are most likely to hear and be heard, stand in one place, vary the height from which you are calling or listening, and turn systematically, calling several times in each direction, then stopping to wait for an answer before turning and calling again, until you've made a full circle. If you walk around while you're trying to call out, your voice won't be as strong and it won't be coming from one place long enough for the person you're calling to find you, even if you're heard. If you walk around while you're trying to listen, you'll be more likely to hear the sound of your own labored breathing than the voice of the person you're trying to find.

Many families who enroll in my Family Protection Training courses go on to ask for private lessons. One such family was planning a vacation in London and then Frankfurt, Germany, and wanted me to train them as a unit. I began with a program I call KNOW & GO, which teaches children to associate particular sounds with proper and safe movements. They learn to identify and respond appropriately to sounds such as cars screeching, smoke alarms, and the phrases pedophiles use to lure their victims.

In London, the mother was window-shopping with her youngest daughter and, at one point, suggested that they cross the street. The child stepped forward, paused, and then said "NO" and pulled the mother back. Just as she did that, a taxi came screeching around the corner, from what for Americans would be the "wrong" direction, and nearly ran them over. The mother looked at her daughter and asked in amazement, "How did you know?" "Mr. Patire taught me to step, stop, and listen," she said, "and that's what I did. That's how I heard the tires screeching." When my client called me on her cell phone to thank me, I told her to thank her daughter for paying such good attention in class.

We're bombarded daily with all kinds of sounds, but learning to distinguish between good sounds and those that are potentially dangerous can help to save your life.

CHECKLIST FOR ACCURATE HEARING

✔ Control your breathing and keep your mind concentrated on what you're doing.

✔ Raise or lower your height so that your voice is pitched to the level of the person you want to hear you, or whom you want to hear.

✔ To increase your "audible zone," change the height from which you're calling and/or listening.

✔ Stand still while you're calling or listening. Don't try to walk and call or walk and listen at the same time.

✔ Systematically change directions and height levels as you're listening and calling out.

✔ Call clearly at least five times in one direction and make sure you pause between each call, then listen for at least ten seconds, and call out and listen again before changing direction.

✔ When you're listening, concentrate on the pitch of the voice you're trying to hear, rather than on actual words. You're much more likely to recognize the tone of a family member's voice than you are to hear what he's saying.

Smell

Each of us has a unique smell, a natural scent that's part of our genetic makeup. In addition, our bodies emanate unique odors not only as a result of perspiration but because of what we've been eating or drinking, if we've been smoking, or where we work. And many people habitually wear a particular perfume, cologne, powder, or aftershave that we come to recognize as uniquely their own. We're all programmed to react to scents that are either particularly pleasing or particularly unpleasant. And particular odors will trigger for each of us particular sensory memories.

Obviously our sense of smell can alert us to a fire or to a noxious chemical in the air. The reason carbon monoxide can be so lethal is that it has no discernible smell. And the gas in our stoves has an odor added to it just so we'll be able to detect a leak. But training ourselves to be aware of what we smell can also provide all-important clues, whether we're looking for a lost loved one or for the perpetrator of a crime. Smell lingers in the air, on clothing, and on other materials. If we can recall and describe a particular odor's having been present at the time of a crime—perhaps the smell of marijuana or cigarettes, even garlic or onions—we might be providing just the piece of information law-enforcement officials need to find the Bad Guy. And if we can describe the perfume or another identifying scent a family member was wearing when he or she disappeared, it might make it easier to find him.

When I was a kid, my father and my uncle Cido used to take my brother and me to stay at their friend Mr. Saulino's farm in upstate New York. One day, during one of those trips, my father, my brother, and I decided to take a walk in the woods while Uncle Cido stayed back at the farmhouse to cook dinner. Before we left, my father asked him what he was making, and my uncle said he was going to cook a sausage dish with peppers, potatoes, and fresh cloves of garlic.

My brother and I were never afraid of anything so long as we were with our father. Dad was a stocky, well-built man who could take care of himself in any situation and whose physical presence alone gave him an air of authority. That day, as we got deeper and deeper into the forest, my brother Tim asked if we could walk along the stream. My father agreed, and before we knew it we'd lost track of time and it was getting dark. I asked my father if he knew his way back and he just smiled and said, "You and your brother wait right here." He then walked about twenty-five yards away and climbed up on a rock, where he stood with his nose in the air, turning in different directions. At one point he stopped and motioned for us to come to him. "Grab my hands," he said, "and come with me." Every hundred or so feet he would put his nose in the air again and then adjust our direction, and before you knew it, we were approaching the farmhouse. As we got closer, we could smell the aroma of the food Uncle Cido was cooking. When we walked in my dad said, "Thanks to your garlic, we made it home in time for dinner." Uncle Cido asked him what he meant, but my dad just touched his finger to his lips and then said, "We'll talk later."

We never discussed the incident again, but many years later when I was traveling overseas on a protection assignment, I asked my father, who had traveled all over when he was in the military, if there was any advice he would give someone going to a strange land. He sat me down and said, "Just remember smell. Smell can be an avenue to your safety, especially if you're lost or it's dark and you can't see where you're going." "What exactly do you mean?" I asked. "Well, Tom," he said, "do you remember when Uncle Cido was alive and we stayed at Mr. Saulino's farmhouse?" "Of course," I said, "those were some of the best times of my life." "Well," he continued, "do you remember the time we were walking in the woods and it was getting dark? You asked me if we were lost, and I said no. Well, we were lost, and if you remember, I climbed up on a rock to get the scent of Uncle Cido's famous sausage dish. I knew how to get home because I followed the scent. The stronger the scent, the closer we were to home. So, when you're in an unfamiliar place, take a good whiff of a unique scent in the air and process that scent as a direction marker. All countries have distinct looks and distinct smells."

My dad was right about smell, as he was about many other things, and that particular safety tip has helped me out on many occasions.

CHECKLIST FOR USING YOUR SENSE OF SMELL

✔ Notice and commit to memory any smell that is distinctive to your family members. If you don't know the name of a cologne, perfume, aftershave, powder, or deodorant someone is using, ask—and remember it.

✔ If you're out with children, remember the smell of what they might have eaten or drunk—orange juice, milk, soda, chocolate, gum, popcorn, french fries, all have distinct odors that might linger on little hands or clothing—especially if something has spilled.

✔ When you're out in areas where there are large groups of people, take note of the smell in the air and around the people who are closest to you.

✔ Should you smell marijuana or alcohol, find out where it's coming from and stay away from those people.

✔ When using your sense of smell to locate someone, try to stay downwind to maximize your chances of picking up a scent.

✔ To enhance your sense of smell, close your eyes and take a deep breath. Let your mind rather than your eyes determine the scent. Our eyes can and do play tricks on our other senses.

LEARNING YOUR ROLES ON THE FAMILY PROTECTION TEAM

Although every adult needs to train his or her senses to be alert for signs of danger, in a Family Protection unit, it's the role of Security to focus on the surroundings and destination as well as to act as the family's protector; make himself known to anyone who might be watching; and initiate the distraction techniques that will provide the Blanket with the window he or she needs to shield the family—particularly children—from danger and evacuate them from the danger site. Remember that it's the role of the Blanket to provide a comfort zone for children and distract them from focusing on an upsetting situation.

The reason for assigning roles to particular members of the team is twofold. First, it's a physical fact that the body responds more quickly and efficiently when it can concentrate on one specific task and follow it through from beginning to end. Second, if more than one person is trying to perform the same task, other members of the team will become confused about whom they should respond to. Make sure that you choose and/or assign roles that play to each person's strength and will therefore afford him or her the greatest level of comfort in a stressful or pressured situation.

ASSIGNING APPROPRIATE ROLES

Generally speaking, the male parent takes the role of Security since he is usually the stronger and better able to protect himself in a potentially violent situation. The female would more naturally serve as the Blanket, protecting and evacuating the children. In situations where there are two males or two females, the adults should work out between them which roles they will take on. The two of you should know each other well enough to make the best decision.

TOM'S TIP

"LOOK OVER THERE!":
THE KEYS TO SUCCESSFUL DISTRACTION

Distraction techniques can be either verbal or physical, or a combination of the two. They involve the use of preplanned statements or movements designed to open a window of opportunity for escape. Sometimes that window can literally be a lifesaver.

Statements that involve references to children make good choices for verbal distraction. Even the most hardened criminal is likely to think twice about harming a child or about harming an adult in the presence of a child. That moment's "second thought" is just the extra few seconds the Blanket might need to get the children out of harm's way. Commands like "Don't touch my baby!" or "Get your hands off my child!" work well in most situations, and they can be accompanied by normal physical actions such as clutching the child close to you. The aggressor is likely to see this as a natural reaction, and it will be easier for the Blanket to initiate cover and evacuation techniques if the child is already within your grasp.

Timing is key to any kind of distraction, and once you've set the technique in motion, there's no turning back. You'll have alerted the aggressor or Bad Guy that you're aware of his intentions, which will trigger a response on his part. But rather than hesitating to set the technique in motion, remember that it's better to evacuate your family unnecessarily than to risk putting them in danger.

On one occasion, my wife asked if I would accompany her and our son to the mall to do some shopping. Of course, being a good, safety-conscious husband, I said yes. As the Security for my family, I'd be able to keep our son occupied and keep an eye on our surroundings while my wife was free to shop. As we were walking through the mall, I noticed two groups of teenagers breakdancing directly in the path where we were walking. As we approached the area they started to congregate around us, so I shuffled my son to my wife and stepped in front of them to take their focus off my family and put it directly on me. As I made eye contact with one of the boys, he shouted, "Hey man, you got a problem, what's the matter, you don't like our dancing?" Because he was about three feet away, I turned and whispered to my wife, "Victoria's Secret." She immediately grabbed our son and walked him away gently but briskly. I picked Victoria's Secret both because it's a woman- and child-friendly store and because it's generally memorable for the lingerie displayed in its windows, and would be easy for security or the police to find, should calling for help become necessary. Mean-

WHAT IF YOU'RE ALONE?

If you're a single parent or simply out alone with your child, what you need to remember is that your first responsibility is to be sure the child is safe. It's your alertness, clearheadedness, and proper decision-making that will keep her that way.

Don't tell your child to "run" unless he is trained to know how and where to run, as we teach in our CDT Family Protection courses. Otherwise he might just run into greater danger.

Do teach your child to move behind you and hold on to you. Make sure you shield his vital areas as well as his line of sight.

If you're near a vestibule or a recessed doorway, tell your child to tuck down next to the wall, and then shield the area with your body.

When I explain to my son how to hold on to me, his mother, or an object, I have him use what I call "Sticky Hands" and demonstrate what I mean by showing him how glue works. Then I play a little game where he becomes Sticky Boy, the newest superhero, and because he believes in superheroes, he likes the concept and practices even when we're just having fun together.

TOM'S TIP

while I stood my ground, and the teenager decided to confront me. He put his finger in my face and said, "Man, what's your problem?" I looked past his eyes as I scanned the others in the group, not saying a word. He made a few more remarks, at which point I stared directly into his eyes, keeping my face expressionless. He backed off and returned to his group as I turned and went to join my family, using the reflection in a store window to keep the teenagers in sight until I was sure there was no longer any danger. When my wife asked what had happened, I simply said, "No big deal, just playing it safe!"

Notice that in this situation my wife and I worked as a team. I acted as Security and took charge. My tone of voice when I said "Victoria's Secret" instantly alerted her to the urgency of the situation, and she immediately protected and evacuated the child without the need for any further communication between us. Happily, nothing happened, but it's possible that without my immediate intervention the situation might have deteriorated into a shoving match or worse.

CHECKLIST FOR EFFECTIVE DISTRACTION

✔ Know when and how to use distraction techniques. The "when" will be your judgment call. You might hear or see something in particular that sets off your internal alarm, or you might just sense that something isn't right. Being in tune with your senses will allow you to trust your own instincts.

✔ Trained actions are always more effective than random actions, so practice, practice, practice.

✔ When you're speaking, don't act; when you're acting, don't speak. The body and mind can really only concentrate fully on one thing at a time. Knowing this, and realizing that both the body and the mind are quick to panic in a potentially dangerous situation, I teach my students that it's imperative for them to concentrate on one specific action at a time. If it's verbal defusion, then think before you talk. If it's action, then think first and act with confidence. Trying to do two things at once will only delay both processes, which might hurt your chances of getting out of the situation unharmed.

✔ Rehearse the specific language you'll be using in your verbal techniques so that your family—particularly the person designated the Blanket—will recognize them immediately.

✔ Timing is key. Once you begin, there's no turning back. Think safety and act safely!

"LET'S GET OUT OF HERE!": COVER AND EVACUATION

Cover and evacuation is, as I've said, the role of the Blanket, who must be alert to the signals being sent by Security, so that she is prepared to do her part to execute the "play" her teammate has put in motion.

Cover and evacuation depends on patterned, practiced movement. "Cover" works on the principle that certain movements can disguise other movements. So cover is, in itself, a kind of distraction.

The first step toward cover and evacuation is shielding the child. Put your body in front of his to form what I call the "protection umbrella." If the child is small, you can guide him into a turn with a slight pressure on his shoulder. If he's slightly bigger, grab the outsides of both his shoulders and turn him gently but firmly. The key to initiating cover and evacuation is to get the child turned away from the danger as quickly as possible and to protect his body with yours.

An important aspect of the Blanket's job is to shield the child from seeing or, if possible, even being aware of violence or danger. Children are very impressionable, and while they might well be too young to understand exactly what's going on, that's all the more reason why they will certainly be left with unpleasant, scary images and lingering fears. If you and your family have the misfortune to be in the wrong place at the wrong time, the following checklist will help to mitigate any potential trauma to your children.

CHECKLIST FOR COVERING AND EVACUATING THE "GIFT"

✔ If you see a violent or potentially volatile situation occurring at some distance, avoid it at all costs. Never stop to watch. Back away from the situation and take an alternate route.

✔ If violence occurs within your children's direct line of sight, pick them up and move them away. If you're with another adult, he or she should step between you and the situation to obstruct their view. If you're alone, shield their view as best you can while escorting them away.

✔ Before offering any explanation of your own, ask your children what they saw. Otherwise you might inadvertently and unnecessarily mention details they hadn't even noticed.

✔ If your children witness a grave act of violence, remove them
as quickly as possible to a place that's familiar and comfortable—
preferably your home. Once you're there, ask them what they saw
or heard before you decide what action will be necessary to guide
them through the experience.

In the aftermath of any violent or frightening situation, it's most
important that you give your children a lot of love, physical comfort, and support. Psychological studies have shown that if a child
witnesses a grave act of violence and if it isn't discussed or explained, the child may develop deep-rooted problems that affect
the course of her entire life. Never underestimate how much children might have understood about, or been affected by, what happened.

Be aware, too, that much of what I've said about actual violence
also applies to acts of violence the child might have seen on television or in the movies. I remember particularly that after the attacks
of September 11, child psychiatrists reminded us that young children are not always able to understand the concept of a taped re-
play and may think the same act is being repeated over and over
again. So be alert to what your child may be viewing.

KNOW YOUR SAFETY ZONES

Knowing your safety zones doesn't mean being afraid to venture
beyond your immediate neighborhood. It means that wherever you
are, you need to be aware and make note of where it's safe for you
to go should you have to find a place to ride out a potentially dangerous situation. Otherwise you might think you're safely evacuating your family when in fact you've just whisked them out of the
frying pan only to put them directly into the fire.

I was once assigned to protect a high-profile family during their
vacation. One day I went with my client's wife and children to a
busy local park where several groups of people were picnicking,
playing ball, tossing a Frisbee, and generally doing what people do

on a nice, sunny day in the park. Suddenly an altercation broke out on the soccer field between two groups of adults who seemed to be vying for "bragging rights." When the fight escalated to the point where one of the men ran to his car and grabbed a gun, I sprang into action.

Because of where we were and where the fight was taking place, we couldn't get back to our car without putting ourselves at risk, so I moved my clients into the women's bathroom, which I'd determined would be our safest bet should the guy decide to start shooting. Luckily, on that occasion the police arrived and broke up the fight before any shots were fired or anyone got hurt, but the point is that you can never know when an unexpected event—one that may have nothing at all to do with you—might put you and your family in danger.

Safety zones are everywhere; you just need to know how to recognize them. If you're on a city street, look for libraries, banks, office buildings, or restaurants, many of which employ security personnel who will be able to help you. Shops also make good safety zones, but those that cater to an adult clientele are better than those that cater to young people. Stores catering to adults tend to hire salespeople who are older and more mature, and who are therefore more likely to respond quickly and calmly when they see that someone's in trouble.

In residential areas, look for well-maintained houses with lights on to indicate that someone is at home. People who care about the upkeep of their homes are most likely to be those who will respond positively to a stranger reporting danger in their neighborhood.

If you're familiar with the neighborhood, check to see if the lights are on in the homes of people you know, and if their cars are in the driveway. Notice whether or not there's any activity inside by glancing in the windows as you pass.

If you begin to practice looking for safety zones every time you're out, it will soon become second nature. And remember that in any potentially dangerous situation, it's always better to retreat to a safe place than to let your pride get in the way of your better judgment and risk getting hurt. "He who runs away will live to run another day" is the motto I teach all my clients.

CHECKLIST FOR FINDING YOUR SAFETY ZONES

✔ Remember that safety zones are everywhere. In commercial areas, look for public buildings that are likely to employ security personnel.

✔ In shopping malls, look for stores that cater to adult women.

TEACHING YOUR CHILD ABOUT SAFETY ZONES

1. First explain to your child what a safety zone is, and why it's important that she know how to find one.

2. Walk her through your neighborhood both during the day and at night, and point out houses that are well lit. Explain how to spot houses that are well kept as well as those that are neglected. Show her which houses belong to people you know and which ones belong to strangers. Make sure the neighbors you choose to point out are ones you know to be trustworthy.

3. Take your child for a ride in unfamiliar but safe neighborhoods both during the day and at night, and let him point out to you the houses that seem well lit and/or well maintained, based on what you've already shown him closer to home. Do the same with businesses, food establishments, libraries, and schools that are both familiar and unfamiliar. Point out that banks, grocery stores, shops that cater to women, toy shops, restaurants, and places of worship are all likely to be good safety zones. Explain to him that, in addition to police stations, firehouses, and hospitals, buildings where there are children and/or adults who work with children are the best safety zones.

4. Point out people of various ages and explain which ones will be more or less likely to keep him safe. Teenagers, for example, are less likely to be child-friendly than senior citizens, who will probably be both more attentive and more responsible.

TOM'S TIP

✔ In familiar residential areas, notice whether people you know are at home. Look for lights, activity, and cars in driveways.

✔ In unfamiliar residential areas, look for well-maintained homes with lights on and activity in or around them.

✔ Practice looking for safety zones until it becomes a part of your daily routine.

HITTING THE ROAD SAFELY

Whether you're taking mass transportation, riding in your own car, or traveling on foot, there are precautions you can and should take to minimize risks to yourself and your family. Certainly, when you're driving you have more control over vehicular safety than you do when you're taking a bus or train, but public transportation is statistically extremely safe. The potential problems are more likely to be created by your fellow travelers. When you're on foot, particularly in unfamiliar places, following certain guidelines will help to ensure your safety while you're exploring or enjoying the scenery.

Riding with Strangers: What You Should Know About Buses, Trains, and Subways

People react differently to traveling in enclosed, often crowded spaces, and it's important that you be aware not only of your own thought processes, but also of the way those around you are behaving. If you notice someone nearby acting in a way that indicates he or she is in some way disturbed, your instinct would be to move away—and that would, of course, be the safest thing to do. But too many of us, when we board a bus, train, or subway, become lost in our own thoughts—what we have to do that day, what we forgot to do before we left, what phone calls we need to make, what we're going to stop and buy for dinner, what we're going to watch on television that evening—almost anything except what's going on around us, and that's when we become likely targets for victimization.

THE UPS AND DOWNS OF SAFETY

Escalators

My son, Tommy, loves escalators, and my wife and I let him ride them as much as possible. Just seeing how much fun he's having gives us pleasure as well. But we also know that escalators can be hazardous; children can get little feet or tiny fingers as well as loose clothing caught in the mechanism. We make sure that whether we're going up or down, one of us is always in front of him to gently lift him off so that he doesn't trip or get a foot stuck in the lip.

Even adults, however, are not immune to accidents on the moving stairs. Escalators in airports or train stations are particularly dangerous because you're often trying to maneuver on and off while carrying your hand luggage, which often leaves you without any way to hold on to the railing. And in crowded arenas or subways, one person reaching the top or the bottom of the flight and not moving out quickly enough can cause a pileup of bodies with nowhere to go.

Elevators

Aside from the possibility that one might break down while you're on it, elevators would appear to be relatively safe. But when they're crowded, as in an office building at rush hour, the unwary rider could easily get stuck in a door or trip over a briefcase or some other object stashed out of sight on the floor. And with backpacks now the preferred way to carry heavy books, not only a child but also a shorter adult is in danger of being smacked in the face. When getting in or out of a crowded elevator, keep an eye on the ground and, if necessary, a hand in front of your face. If you're riding with a child, remember that it can be even more dangerous down there than it is at your eye level, and try to create a shield of safety for the little one. Hold on to the child so that you don't get separated if the doors should close, and don't worry about being the first one in or out; it's not worth getting pushed or crushed, and there will always be another elevator. Never use your child's stroller as a wedge to prevent the door from closing. If the safety mechanism should fail, your child would be caught and possibly injured.

Tom's Elevator Tips

- Keep a firm grip on your purse or wallet. Crowded elevators are among pickpockets' favorite workplaces.

- Always scan to see who's in the elevator before you get on. If anyone looks suspicious, wait for the next one.

- If you're alone in the elevator and someone gets in who sets off your internal alarm, try to get out right away.

- If you can't get out, stand with your back to the wall and concentrate on the door, but keep your eye on the one who made you suspicious. Don't engage in conversation and do get off at the next stop, whether or not it's your floor.

- Realistically, being assaulted in the elevator of a reputable hotel or office building is unlikely because the assailant is so likely to get caught. If the worst should happen, however, and you're involved in an assault or an attempted rape, try to hit all the buttons as you struggle.

- Try to wedge yourself into a corner with your back to the wall and hold the assailant off with your hands and feet.

- If the assailant hits the "stop" button, an alarm will go off, and in most cases, help will be on the way.

Stairways

Rushing and not holding on to the railing are two of the most frequent causes of stairway accidents. If you're rushing, you could easily trip or slip and cause yourself serious injury. If someone else is rushing and bumps into you or pushes past you, you could also find yourself tumbling head over heels, particularly if you weren't holding on. If you're carrying packages, your view might be impeded. And if you're carrying a child, you need to be particularly careful because losing your footing will mean falling either on or with that child. If you're climbing with a child who's walking, keep him in front of you to prevent his falling backwards. If you're descending, walk in front of the child and set a slow pace, stopping every few steps to be sure he's not lagging behind.

The crimes most often associated with mass transportation are purse snatchings, pickpocketing, and thefts of items like laptop computers or gold chains. Most of these occur when the vehicle is stopping and people are getting on and off, because the jostling and activity provide excellent cover for thieves. People are most likely to be targeted when they are entering or exiting, sitting in aisle seats, or standing; other likely targets are those who are simply unsuspecting and easily distracted. The Bad Guy might use a prop such as a garment carried in one hand or thrown over his arm or shoulder to shield his movements and hide the item once it is taken. Very often, because the victim isn't paying attention and the thief is so good at his job, the person who is robbed doesn't even know when it's happening.

Whenever you're in a public space, particularly in a crowded, small space like a bus, a train, or a subway car, it's important to remain in the moment and be alert to what's going on around you.

My friend Mike told me a story that illustrates just how important this can be. Mike commutes from Hoboken to his job in Manhattan on the same train every day. After traveling this route for several months, he became familiar with many of the other commuters whom he saw on a daily basis. One sunny morning he noticed a well-dressed man he'd never seen before enter the train carrying a long trenchcoat. The gentleman sat down next to a woman who was also dressed in what was obviously business attire, and lay his coat down between them. At the next stop, just as the doors were beginning to close, he jumped up, exclaiming, "Oh, this is my stop," and hastily made his way out. Nobody thought anything of it because many commuters are preoccupied and it isn't unusual for someone to almost miss his or her stop. At the next stop, however, as the woman he'd been sitting next to stood up preparing to exit, she suddenly shouted, "My purse, my purse, its been stolen!"

When Mike told me about the incident, I knew that the man with the coat had been a true professional. The problem with our society is that we believe people who rob or steal ought to look strange or unkempt, while, in reality, they're usually well-groomed individuals who make sure they don't stick out in a crowd.

CHECKLIST FOR MASS TRANSIT SAFETY

✔ When entering or exiting, keep a tight grip on your purse, briefcase, laptop, or other hand luggage, and, if the strap is long enough, wrap it around your wrist for additional security.

✔ If possible, choose a seat by the window rather than on the aisle, and place your purse or briefcase between you and the window, where it will be harder to grab.

✔ If you're taking a nap, wrap your arms around your purse or briefcase or put your case on the floor wedged between your feet and the window, where it will be not only harder to reach but also out of sight. Put your wallet in the front pocket of your pants on the side closest to the window, or put it in your inside jacket pocket and cross your arms for added protection.

✔ If you do have to sit near the aisle, keep your belongings on your lap, wrapped in your arms.

✔ To thwart would-be pickpockets, keep your wallet in a front trousers pocket or the inside pocket of your jacket, never in a back pants pocket or an outside jacket pocket.

✔ Keep gold chains and other necklaces tucked inside your shirt, blouse, or sweater, where they'll be out of sight to a thief. To make yourself a less likely target, remove flashy rings, watches, and earrings before boarding. You can always put them on again when you reach your destination. "Out of sight, out of mind" holds very true in this case.

✔ If standing is your only option, hold on to the bar or strap with one hand and keep the other hand firmly on your purse or briefcase. Be alert to people pushing past you as they enter or exit.

✔ Wherever you are—sitting or standing—continuously scan your surroundings (remember: left to right). Not only will you be more likely to spot potential trouble before it occurs, but potential troublemakers will see that you're alert and aware and will take their trouble elsewhere.

✔ If a stranger asks you a question, be brief but polite. If the approach is meant to distract you while an accomplice picks your pocket, you don't want to give him that time; and if the questioner is in any way disturbed, you don't want to trigger a confrontation by appearing to be rude.

✔ Whenever you travel with a child, put her in an inside seat with you on the aisle as protection. Or, if you must stand, keep the child in front of you, where your body will protect her from the crowd and you'll be able to hold on to her and prevent her from falling.

When You're in the Driver's Seat

Assuming that you're a safe driver, and that both you and your passengers wear your seatbelts at all times, your greatest risks when driving (aside from other drivers) occur because you've neglected to take the simple precautions that would ensure the safety of your vehicle, such as checking the fuel gauge, the oil, or the radiator fluid.

Even in a worst-case scenario, however, cars don't often break down to the point where they can't be driven at all. If you should break down in an unfamiliar or isolated area, try to get to a public location like a mall or a gas station. If you can't do that, pull as close to the curb or as far onto the shoulder of the road as you can, to minimize your risk of being hit by another driver. Put on your hazard lights and stay inside your vehicle.

These days it would be foolish for anyone ever to get in a car without a fully charged cell phone, but if you don't have one, try to watch for public phones so that you'll be able to locate one should you need it. And if you're traveling with children, never, under any circumstances, leave them alone in the car while you go for help.

CHECKLIST FOR SAFE DRIVING

✔ Check your spare tire regularly to be sure that both the tire and the equipment needed to change it are in good working order.

✔ Always keep a well-stocked first-aid kit in your car.

GOOD SAMARITANS AND ROADSIDE HELP

If you're stuck on the side of the road, and a "good Samaritan" stops to offer help, be cautious.

- Stay in your car. Above all, don't try to hitch a ride.
- Ask him to call a tow truck or the police.
- Never accept the offer of a ride to the nearest gas station.

If you see someone in need of help, you still need to be cautious.

- If there are children in your car, get the attention of the person in trouble and indicate—without getting out of your car—that you are calling for help.
- If someone really seems desperate and you're on a major road, in broad daylight, with plenty of traffic, you might decide to stop. Sometimes you just have to use your best judgment.
- Never, under any circumstances, stop to pick up a hitchhiker.
- Selfish or not, when you're deciding whether or not to stop and help, always consider your own welfare first.

TOM'S TIP

✔ Make sure a flashlight and extra batteries are in the car at all times.

✔ Always carry a fully charged cell phone with an extra charged battery and an adapter that plugs into your car's cigarette lighter. If you don't already own a cell phone, I would strongly suggest that you buy one for just such an emergency, but, in the meantime, keep spare change in the glove compartment, the console, or the ashtray (assuming you don't smoke in the car) to use if you have to make a call.

✔ Program emergency numbers into your cell phone.

✔ Always check the fuel gauge before putting your car into motion.

✔ Keep a quart of oil, a gallon of water, a can of tire-fixer, a charged spare battery, and other items for a quick emergency repair in the trunk of your car at all times.

✔ Keep a selection of maps in your vehicle just in case you find yourself in an unfamiliar area with no friendly faces to give you directions.

The most dangerous times for drivers may be when they're not on the road at all, but when they're entering and leaving their cars. There are, however, precautions you can take to reduce the chances that you'll become a victim in such situations.

CHECKLIST FOR PARKING SAFETY

✔ Always park as close to your destination as possible, even if it means waiting a few minutes for a space to become available.

✔ When it's dark, try to park under a streetlight or in a well-lit area.

✔ In a parking lot, back into the parking space so that you'll be facing forward and able to drive away quickly if necessary.

✔ Leave the engine running until you've gathered all your belongings, so that you'll be able to get out of the car as soon as the engine is off. Survey your surroundings before you open the door.

✔ Remove or hide all valuables before leaving the car.

✔ Take the best-lit route from the car to your destination.

✔ When returning to your car, have your keys in your hand so that you can get in quickly or use them as a weapon if necessary. Take the best-lit route and survey the area around your vehicle from a distance before you approach. Walk one car length past yours and circle around it so that you have a clear view of everything in and around the car before you approach it.

✔ Once you've opened the doors, check both front and back seats to be certain no one is lurking inside before you or any members of your family get in.

✔ Once you're inside, lock all the doors immediately.

✔ If you are approached by an assailant, call attention to yourself by honking your horn and flashing your lights.

✔ If you have any sense of danger when parking or returning to your car, follow your instincts. Retreat to the nearest safety zone until you're sure the area is secure, or call the police.

In addition to maximizing your own safety, following the rules above and installing an alarm or a built-in immobilizing system will also help to ensure that your car isn't stolen while it's parked. It ought to go without saying that you should never leave a set of keys in the car, even if you think they're hidden in the glove box. Approximately 20 percent of all vehicle thefts involve keys left in the car, at a valet box, or in the pocket of a checked coat.

Carjacking

Returning from dinner or a shopping expedition to discover that your car has been stolen is certainly unpleasant, inconvenient, even frightening, but it isn't life-threatening. Carjacking is another issue entirely. If it's a question of you or your car, get out and give it up. Unfortunately, however, most carjackers won't take the time to give you that option. And if there's a child or an elderly person in the car with you, the question of whether you can get him or her out or whether you should stay and try to protect your loved one, both complicates the problem and increases the danger that someone will get hurt. Most carjackings occur because the vehicle is simply in the wrong place at the wrong time, and there are precautions you can take to minimize the chances that you and your car will be targeted.

Not long ago, I was at a seminar where I met a martial arts instructor who told me the following story about how he was carjacked. He'd been driving home after teaching class at about ten o'clock on a Friday night. He stopped at a convenience store to buy a bottle of water and then continued on his way. When he turned in to a side street, he saw another car behind him. The driver was flashing his lights and waving rather frantically out the window, indicating that he should pull over. Thinking it might be one of his students, he pulled to the curbside. As soon as he did that, two male teenagers approached either side of his car. When he asked what was going on, the one closest to him pulled out a gun and told him to put his wallet on the passenger seat and get out of the car. When he looked across at the teenager on the passenger side, he saw that he, too, had a gun. Being a smart man, he stepped out of the car and followed their directions. They then told him to go sit on the curb on the other side of the street. As he was moving in the direction they'd indicated, they jumped in his car and took off. Neither his car nor his valuables were ever recovered, but because he'd followed directions, he got out of the situation unharmed.

CHECKLIST FOR CARJACKING PREVENTION

✔ Avoid driving in isolated areas.

✔ If you're traveling an unfamiliar route, check and recheck directions before you set out, so that you don't have to pull over and stop along the way.

✔ Be alert to what's happening on the road around you.

✔ Don't tailgate. Carjackers love to box you in and not leave you any way out. So, if you tailgate, you're doing half their work for them. All the carjackers have to do is pull up alongside and steer you in whatever direction they want. If you're boxed in with no way to escape, you're theirs!

✔ Whenever possible, drive in the middle lane to minimize the chance of being forced off the road by another vehicle.

✔ If you are stopped in traffic, be sure to leave enough room between your car and the one in front of you to make a quick departure. One full car length will generally provide the room you need.

✔ If you are carjacked, don't struggle, and pay attention to what the carjacker is telling you. If you're alone, and you're given the opportunity, get out and get away. If there are vulnerable passengers in the car, such as a child or a senior citizen, you'll have to make a hard decision about the best course of action. Try to remain calm so that you'll be able to think more clearly, difficult as that may be. My suggestion would be to tell the carjacker you don't want any trouble because your child or your mother (or whoever is in the car with you) has a medical condition and you're going to take him/her out of the car. Most carjackers don't want trouble, either; they just want your vehicle, and, in fact, it's rare for a carjacker to target a driver with passengers in the car.

✔ If you see another driver flashing his lights as an indication for you to pull over, go to a public area such as a convenience store or a strip mall to minimize your chances of being carjacked.

SAFE STROLLING

One of the best and most pleasurable ways to explore unfamiliar territory is to walk around and see the sights, but it's also when we're on unfamiliar ground that we need to be the most cautious and alert to our surroundings.

Several years ago, clients of mine were vacationing in Acapulco. One evening they went dancing at a local disco and decided that instead of taking a taxi back to the hotel, they'd go for a moonlight stroll. As they turned a corner onto a deserted street, they were met by a gentleman who identified himself as a police officer, although he wasn't in uniform and didn't offer any form of identification (nor did my clients ask to see any). The "officer" told them it wasn't a good idea to be walking these streets and suggested that if they crossed the road they'd not only be safer but also would have a better view of the ocean.

My clients thanked him politely and did as he'd suggested. They'd gone no more than a hundred yards farther when they were accosted by two young men who robbed them at gunpoint, relieving them of all their valuables as well as their shoes (no doubt to ensure that they wouldn't be chased on foot). When they tried to flag down a passing cab for help, the driver only laughed at them, and it wasn't until another tourist in a taxi made his driver stop that they received any assistance.

When they told him about the incident, the concierge at their hotel only shrugged and said that was why they'd been asked not to leave the premises. And, because the thieves had made off with their passports along with their valuables, they had to make a trip to the American embassy and their return home was delayed for four days while they waited for new passports.

CHECKLIST FOR WALKING IN SAFETY

All of the following precautions also apply to power walking, jogging, cycling, or any other form of outdoor exercise you engage in by yourself.

✔ Plan ahead and know your final destination. Don't just "wander."

✔ If possible, wear shoes and clothing that allow for ease of movement. Tight clothing and uncomfortable shoes will restrict the speed with which you are able to get away if necessary.

✔ Keep jewelry and other valuables out of sight.

✔ Walk confidently, with your head held high and your body erect. Try to stay close to the curb, particularly when buildings are screened by shrubbery, in dark alleys, or in other poorly lit areas.

✔ Always be alert and aware of your surroundings.

✔ Scan the distance as well as your immediate surroundings so that you don't inadvertently wander into a danger zone. Trust your instincts and avoid any area you think might be unsafe.

✔ At night, keep to well-lit areas and wear reflective tape on the front, back, and sides of your outer garment (or purchase a special reflective vest designed for walkers, runners, and cyclists, available in many sporting goods stores).

✔ On the road, always walk facing oncoming traffic.

✔ Use reflective surfaces such as mirrors or windows to check what's behind and across from you. If you suspect you're being followed, head for the nearest safety zone. Should someone try to accost you from a vehicle, try to run in the direction opposite to the one in which the vehicle is traveling.

✔ Keep your distance from strangers in order to give yourself more time to act rather than react. Try to remain in control of your emotions so that you'll be able to think more clearly.

✔ Evaluate any advice given to you by a stranger, especially if it's unsolicited. Bad Guys usually work in teams, so the one giving you directions just might be setting you up.

✔ Always have a cover and evacuation plan in place.

STAYING SAFE ON CAMPUS

My older brothers and I were very close growing up, and both of them are now blessed with beautiful daughters for whom I have, naturally enough given my line of work, played the role of concerned and protective uncle. So when my brother Phil's daughter, Dana, was about to enter college, I made it my business to check out her chosen school. I was amazed as I walked through the campus at various times on several different days to see the variety of people rushing to class, talking with one another, or just strolling along. I realized, too, that a campus—virtually any campus—is wide open and accessible to anyone at any time. Some of the people I encountered didn't seem to have any real business being on campus and were just there to enjoy the sights, which in most instances meant the girls rather than the scenery. I myself certainly didn't fit the profile of a college student or professor and yet no one, including the two security officers from whom I asked directions, ever stopped me or questioned my being there. After that experience, I was curious, so I decided to visit several other campuses in the area in order to develop a checklist for campus safety that might help not only my niece but other young women as well.

Thanks to a federal law championed by the parents of a young woman who was murdered on a university campus in 1986, called

CYCLING SAFETY

If you're out riding your bike and a couple of punks want to steal it, let them. You can always get another bike.

It's a different story, however, when children are bike-riding alone. Another kid might want his bike, but an adult approaching a child on a bike usually wants the child, not the bike. Train your child so that if an adult approaches him while he's out riding, he will entwine himself with the bike, making it as difficult as possible for the would-be abductor to separate one from the other. Chances are he's not going to risk being seen struggling to separate a child from a bike, so the more the child struggles to hold on to the bike, the more likely it is that the abductor will give up and move on.

TOM'S TIP

the Jeanne Clery Disclosure of Campus Policy and Campus Crime Statistics Act (commonly known as the Jeanne Clery Act), colleges and universities are required to disclose timely and annual statistics regarding crimes and security policies on their campuses. Most reported crimes fall into one of seven categories: criminal homicide, sex offenses, robbery, aggravated assault, burglary, motor vehicle theft, and arson. What remains unknown, however, is what percentage of incidents go unreported.

While some campus crimes are no different from those in the general population, others—such as hazing, overindulgence in alcohol and drugs, and students exploiting other students—are more directly related to college life. One particularly prevalent type of exploitation occurs when young women are encouraged to become intoxicated and are then raped or photographed in the nude. In many cases, the women don't even know what happened until they or their friends see the photos on a pornographic college website.

I was thankfully able to prevent just that kind of exploitation when, several years ago, a client asked me to provide security for a college party that was to be held at his catering hall. He told me the party-goers would range in age from eighteen to twenty-three and that approximately 200 guests were expected to attend. Knowing how quickly word of a party can spread on campus, I purposely overstaffed for the event and, sure enough, by 10 P.M. there were approximately 400 young men and women at various stages of intoxication in the hall.

Before the evening was over, Colleen, a young woman I knew from the local area, came up to me and said that her friend had passed out and two young men had taken her into the men's room and locked the door. I and one of my staff went to the door and shouted that if they didn't open up, we'd have them arrested. Sure enough, they let us in, and we found the young woman partially undressed on the floor and one of the guys holding a disposable camera, which we immediately confiscated. I asked Colleen to dress her friend and called the police to make a report.

At the end of the evening, Colleen asked us to help get her friend home. We drove them to the friend's house, carried her up the stairs, and laid her on the bed. Then, leaving Colleen to keep an eye on her in case she became sick, we went on our way.

Not too many years later, on a visit to the doctor's office, I was greeted by an attractive young nurse who stared at me for a moment and then asked if I remembered her. I didn't, but it turned out that she was the young woman we'd carried up the stairs that night. "I always wanted to thank you," she said. "I've seen you many times but I was always too embarrassed to approach you." Then she paused and said, "Thank you." She went on to tell me that she no longer drinks and that she still has nightmares about the photographs that were taken that night and what might have been done to her if we hadn't been there to stop it.

CHECKLIST FOR CAMPUS SAFETY

✔ *Know your surroundings.* With an adult along to help defuse any unexpected situation that might arise, walk, drive, and get to know both the campus and the surrounding area before you begin attending classes. The best time to do this is during the summer, when the campus is less populated and the roads are less busy. Do this at night as well as in the daytime so that you know which areas are well lit.

✔ *Get to know your secure zones.* As you walk the campus, make note of well-lit areas as well as the location of security stations and public telephones.

✔ *Screen new acquaintances.* When meeting someone for the first time, engage in limited, polite conversation but don't convey any personal information until you're sure of the person you're dealing with. Should the person be intoxicated, leave as soon as you can do so without antagonizing him. If the person touches you, scream and draw attention to yourself.

✔ *Make sure someone knows where you are.* A parent or a trusted friend or both should be made aware of your schedule, especially if you're attending a meet-and-greet party with a group of strangers. Carrying a cell phone is a good way to stay secure and in touch.

✔ *Travel in groups.* Whenever possible, travel with a group of people. If you're alone, try to find a group of people you know and stay close to them. Coed groups are safer than groups of women, and any group is safer than being alone.

✔ *Know the ins and outs.* Become familiar with all the exits in the buildings where you attend classes in case you need to evacuate quickly. Check to see what kinds of locks there are on the windows on the first and second floors so that you can use them if you have to make an emergency escape.

✔ *Know your visitors.* If you live on or near the campus, don't give out your address until you're certain it's safe to do so. Familiarize yourself with those who live in your dorm or your area, and never, ever, let anyone know where you keep a spare key.

✔ *Be prepared.* Carry on your person or program your cell phone with the numbers of campus security, the dean of students, and, if there is one, the emergency hotline.

✔ *Spotlight your concern.* If you have any concern at all about any aspect of safety, document it with a written report to campus security and the dean of students. The brighter the spotlight you shine on the problem, the quicker it is likely to be addressed. Be sure to follow up to see what is being done, and if you're not satisfied, report your concerns to the college or local newspaper.

✔ *When in doubt, walk on out.* This is the golden rule you should follow at all times. Anyone can find him- or herself in the wrong place at the wrong time. If you're ever at a function or in a group and suspect that something potentially dangerous or of a criminal nature is taking place, leave immediately. Do not risk becoming involved in any activity that could affect your life and your livelihood now or in the future.

✔ *Stay close to your belongings.* If you carry your personal belonging in a backpack or a tote bag as many students do, be sure they are on your person or within your sight at all times. In addition, be sure to carry emergency cash in a pocket to make a quick purchase or to use in an emergency.

SAFETY IN CROWDS

The potential for being trampled by a panic-stricken crowd in places like a nightclub, a sports arena, or a theater is certainly a concern, but learning how to gauge the mood of the crowd and to see the panic coming is, like many other skills, something that one can learn.

First, it's important to understand that the primary concern of businesspeople organizing a concert or a sporting event is to get as many people as possible *into* the venue. In most instances this means that the ratio of security personnel to attendees is far smaller than would be ideal. And yet the percentage of such events that run perfectly smoothly is far greater than the percentage of those that don't.

One event for which I provided security some years ago could have ended in tragedy but luckily did not. It was at one of the most prestigious nightclubs in New Jersey. The place was extremely overcrowded, which meant that those of us providing security had only limited freedom of movement.

Someone in the middle of the crowd whom I can only describe as an incredible jerk decided to give everyone a scare by setting off a large firecracker known as an M-80. The noise was deafening and the crowd immediately panicked. Everyone in the room ran for the front door. There were other exits, some of them even closer, but in their anxiety, no one was able to think of any way out other than the way they'd come in. A waitress was knocked to the ground and trampled by what had quickly turned into a human stampede. I rushed to her aid with one of my men and we moved her out of harm's way. Luckily, because of our training, she suffered no more than a few bruises and was back at work the following week. As she later told me, "One second I was picking up drinks and the next you guys were picking me up."

WHEN MY BROTHERS and I were growing up, my father, the police officer, always made sure to point out the exits at any event or restaurant we went to "just in case." Too many people, however, trust—without any real basis for such belief—that security personnel will ensure their safety at public events, and too often their trust is misplaced.

It's true that the security at high-profile celebrity events has been increased since the terrorist attacks of September 11, 2001. In fact, I had the privilege to be a part of one of the most professional teams ever assembled when I provided security for the Grammy Awards in New York City in 2003. But one can't always count on that level of protection at less public and less highly publicized events, which is why it's important that each individual take responsibility for his or her own safety.

IF YOU'RE CAUGHT IN A MOB

Since no amount of planning can guarantee that things won't go wrong, you might at some time find yourself caught in a crowd that turns into a reckless mob. If that should happen, remember the following:

1. *Curb your curiosity.* It killed the proverbial cat, and it can endanger your life too. Don't waste time trying to see what's going on. Just get yourself and your family to safety as quickly as possible—sometimes even seconds can make a difference.

2. *Move* away *from the center.* The closer you are to the center of the crowd, the more likely it is that you'll be trapped or trampled. Stay on the outside and, if possible, use the walls to guide you toward the nearest exit.

3. *Scan and move.* Keep moving at a steady, urgent pace, constantly scanning from left to right and low to high, looking for fallen objects that might cause you to trip and fall. Don't stop unless you determine that the route you have chosen is blocked, and don't run aimlessly. Moving too quickly may cause you to trip and fall.

4. *Hold on to one another.* If you are traveling with a group, hold on to one another's belts or pant legs, or whatever you can grab to prevent yourselves from being separated.

5. *Pick up your child.* Hold the child securely with his or her chest facing you and try to keep him calm. As you move, keep on yelling, "Child here! Child here!"

6. *Stay calm.* When emotions run high, panic sets in. Try to remain calm and think before you act.

7. *Protect your eyes.* If the room is smoky or chemicals have been released, stay as close to the ground as you can and try to avoid looking directly into the pollutant. Scan at a 45-degree angle and blink frequently to moisturize your eyes. Don't rub your eyes. Your hands may have come in contact with the pollutant, and using them to rub your eyes may just make matters worse.

8. *Stick to your plan.* Once you've decided on an escape route, keep moving toward your goal. Don't stop to second-guess yourself or try to go back for something you think you've forgotten. Whatever you've left behind can be replaced; your life cannot.

9. *If you're knocked down.* Make yourself as small as possible by rolling into a ball, and protect your head and vital organs. If you feel yourself panicking, try to regulate your breathing and gather your thoughts. Get up as quickly as possible, even if it means inching your way to an upright position. If there are other people on top of you, use your hands and forearms to create a breathing space. Take short, steady breaths and try to control your anxiety.

10. *Stay focused.* No matter what happens, stay focused on survival. The key to survival is to never give in to self-pity.

11. *Regroup.* Once you're outside, take a count of the others in your group. If someone is missing, look for a police officer, a security officer, or another able-bodied person and ask for help. Do not go back yourself unless there is absolutely no other alternative.

TOM'S TIP

CHECKLIST FOR SAFETY IN CROWDS

✔ *Know the layout.* As soon as you arrive, scan the venue for all accessible exits, including windows if you happen to be on the ground floor. Look for sprinklers, fire alarms, and fire extinguishers. The more of them there are, the safer you are.

✔ *Talk it over.* Discuss with your companions what you will do if something untoward occurs and you need to evacuate quickly.

✔ *Plan your escape routes.* Work out an escape route and have several backup plans in mind. It's always best to choose an exit that *isn't* in direct sight because the majority of the crowd will rush toward the door they see first.

✔ *Plan your meeting place.* Know in advance where you and your friends or loved ones will meet if you should be separated. Make sure the place you choose is outside the facility where the event is taking place and in a secure, easily accessible location.

✔ *Assess the crowd.* If the group is becoming rowdy, get out as fast as you can—before trouble starts.

✔ *Be proactive, not reactive.* If an alarm goes off, leave immediately. Once you're outside is time enough to determine whether or not it was a false alarm.

AVOIDING THE HAZARDS OF LONG-DISTANCE TRAVEL

People today are more apprehensive about long-distance travel, especially to international destinations, than ever before. As I've said more than once, however, your chances of being involved in a hijacking or a plane or train crash are infinitesimal compared with the much more likely hazards you might experience in an unfamiliar location. Some of us travel frequently on business, while for others getting on a plane usually means vacation. Vacations are supposed to be relaxing and fun, and taking a few precautions can ensure that your fun won't be spoiled.

Although air rage appears to be on the rise, it is generally a Bad Guest rather than a Bad Guy who causes the trouble. Even a Bad Guest can, however, wreak havoc in the sky, as was demonstrated when I was contacted by a gentleman named Kristen L. Skogrand who had been assaulted and suffered injuries as a result of air rage at an altitude of 35,000 feet. He'd been acting as a good Samaritan, trying to protect a fellow passenger who was traveling with children, when the enraged passenger turned on him. Not only was he injured, but other passengers, particularly the children aboard, were severely traumatized, and, perhaps worst of all, the plane was unable to land for more than two hours following the assault.

As a result of his experience, Mr. Skogrand has been inspired to educate others about how to protect themselves in these situations. His website, www.safeflier.com, tells his story in depth and provides some very useful information about what to look for and what to do when one encounters an air rage situation.

In addition to taking basic precautions in the airport and on the plane, it also makes sense to find out as much as you can about the country, city, or other location you're going to be visiting.

When you are in your own country, remember that there are Bad

Guys everywhere and that they're most likely to prey upon someone who looks lost, confused, or who doesn't "fit in." And try not to "get lost" if you possibly can help it. First of all, you might find yourself in an area you don't want to be in, and, second, you might have to ask a stranger—who just might turn out to be a Bad Guy—for directions. To avoid those situations, get directions before you leave your hotel. If you don't trust the staff, call the local police switchboard. Usually, they will not only provide the directions you need but will also give you a brief rundown of the do's and don'ts of their town.

If you're traveling abroad, there may be dress codes, ways of behaving, even laws you're unfamiliar with. In some cultures it would be inappropriate for women to wear trousers or to bare their arms; in others, showing the sole of your shoe is considered offensive. In Singapore, it's against the law to chew gum on the street. Violating an unspoken dress code or engaging in some innocent behavior whose meaning is different in the place you're visiting can make you extremely uncomfortable; violating a law you didn't even know existed, however, can land you in a foreign jail.

If you don't speak the local language, it would be useful to learn a few basic words and phrases that might come in handy and that will certainly endear you to the native population, who will appreciate your having made the effort. Those I usually suggest include the following:

- Hello.
- Good-bye.
- Please.
- Thank you.
- You're welcome.
- What time is it?
- How much does it cost?
- Can you help me?
- Where's the hospital?
- Call the police.

STAY COMFORTABLE AND SAFE
IN THE AIRPORT AND ON THE PLANE

1. Never let your hand luggage or valuables out of your sight, and never ask a stranger to watch them.

2. Never let small children "explore" the airport alone. You might choose to let your teenager go off for a snack, but make sure you have a set time and place to meet afterwards. If you have an extra cell phone, give it to her so that you know you can contact her if she doesn't show up when and where she's supposed to.

3. Even if you're checking your luggage (very often I travel with only what I can carry on), make sure you have a small carry-on bag with snacks, water, and reading material. The heightened security in airports means that waiting has become a way of life, so, instead of becoming frustrated or aggravated, be prepared and spend your time wisely.

4. If you're traveling with children, make sure you have a supply of small games, crayons, and books—whatever it takes to keep them happy rather than cranky while waiting and during the flight.

5. Once you're in your seat, while other passengers are still boarding, remain alert. Notice who boards the aircraft, and let them see that you're paying attention. If you see or hear anything out of the ordinary, alert the flight attendant, not by ringing the call button but by getting up and approaching her discreetly, without calling attention to yourself, when the time is right. Once everyone's on board and settled in, make yourself comfortable and prepare to use your time wisely—whether that means doing work, reading a book, listening to music, or taking a nap.

6. If you're a strong and able-bodied person, let the flight crew know that you're ready and able to help them if they need you. Don't be aggressive about it; just make the suggestion. Airlines have been training the crews to be better prepared for in-flight emergencies, and as one who has consulted with several of them, I know that a key factor in this training is to teach crew members to use their resources wisely. In an emergency situation, a willing and able passenger could become just the additional resource they need.

TOM'S TIP

CHECKLIST FOR SAFE TRAVEL

✔ Research your destination. Find out about climate, culture, customs, and laws.

✔ Check with the U.S. State Department to see if there's a travel advisory in effect.

✔ Pack appropriately for both the meteorological and cultural climate. It's better to blend in than to stand out.

✔ Learn basic phrases in the local language.

✔ Find out what foods and beverages, if any, to avoid.

✔ Bring medications for diarrhea and nausea.

✔ Check the local weather forecasts both before and during your travels.

✔ Be sure to have all the vaccinations required or recommended for your destination.

✔ Attend to all cuts and scrapes immediately, particularly in the tropics, where infection sets in easily.

✔ Bring along some bottled water in case of emergency.

✔ Insect repellent, sunscreen, and hats are a must in hot climates.

✔ Know the location of the American embassy or consulate in the city where you'll be staying.

✔ Enjoy conversing with people, but avoid confrontation. Speaking in generalities is usually the best idea.

✔ Always carry a copy of your passport in addition to the original and in a separate place, just in case the original is lost or stolen.

✔ Enjoy your surroundings, but be aware of what's going on around you and try to keep a low profile rather than standing out.

✔ It's always a good idea to have some money in U.S. dollars as well as traveler's checks, credit cards, and local currency when traveling abroad.

PASSPORT SAFETY

Keep the original on your person—not in a pocketbook or backpack—in a place you check frequently. I keep mine in the inside pocket of my sportcoat, if I'm wearing one, or in a front trouser pocket. You'll need to have the original with you in case you have to show it for any reason. You can carry the copy in your bag or check it in the hotel safe. You can also scan it into your computer and put it into a secure file so that, should you lose it, you can always download a copy.

TOM'S TIP

Being in an unfamiliar location also makes it more difficult to know where it's safe or unsafe to venture on foot. Rio de Janeiro, for example, one of the most beautiful vacation spots on earth, is known for the thieves who prey on foreign visitors, and tourists are warned of the danger.

At home, you know where the "good" and "bad" neighborhoods are, but when you're on holiday it's easy to forget that other cities have good and bad neighborhoods as well. The concierge at your hotel can probably provide you with some useful tips, and you'd do well to take his advice—as my clients in Acapulco discovered when it was too late.

When returning to your hotel from an outing, always use the main entrance and make sure that you're visible. You might, for example, make it a point to ask a question at the front desk so that you know someone on staff has seen you and will remember you, and you will become a less attractive target than an anonymous tourist whom nobody knows.

You'd also do well, however, to remember that hotels are essentially public buildings in which anyone has access to all floors at any time, and employees have keys to every room. Housekeeping and other staff may be poorly paid, and valuables left in your room could well be a temptation. Many hotels provide a safe in every room, and there's always a safe in the lobby. Make use of them. In addition, prospective thieves often get information about guests from hotel employees such as housekeepers, waiters, or those who work poolside. To minimize your chances of being targeted, be cautious about displaying money and jewelry in public.

While the management and staff may want to do all they can to ensure your comfort and safety, you need to take some responsibility as well.

I was once hired to protect a Fortune 500 client who was traveling to a South American country where certain people had good reason to dislike him. When I arrived with my staff, the client had already checked in and retired for the night. The first thing I did after we'd checked in was to ask for him at the desk, and when they gave me his room number, I immediately went to his room, woke him up, and made him move into the room that had been assigned to me. Rule number one in the protection business is never to register a high-profile client under his own or his corporation's name.

Once I knew my client was safely tucked away in my room, I went back to his room with one of my staff. The first thing we did was a bit of judicious furniture moving, just in case we had unexpected guests. Then we went over our plans for the following day and finally got to bed at about two o'clock in the morning. Two hours later I heard our door rattling, and muffled conversation in the hall. I whispered to my partner to get his attention, but he couldn't hear me over the noise of the antiquated air-conditioning system, so I hit him in the head with a pillow instead. At that moment the door flew open and we leaped to our feet, taking cover against the walls. Three male intruders came through the doorway and immediately fell over the two chairs we'd tipped over in front of the entrance as obstacles. As soon as they'd regained their footing, they took off down the hall and into the stairwell.

We didn't bother to chase them. Instead we awakened our other team members and went to check on our client, who was sleeping peacefully. Returning to our room, we found a double-edged knife on the floor between the two chairs.

SLEEPING IN THE GREAT OUTDOORS

Camping is a popular way to spend a family vacation. It can be great fun, but it also means staying alert for animal predators as well as potential human ones. If you decide to take your family camping, here are a few tips to make sure they remain safe:

1. Know the extended weather forecast before you leave, and plan accordingly.

2. Map out your destination, and have two backup routes just in case there's a traffic jam or a road is closed for some unexpected reason.

3. When you arrive at the campsite, check out the area before you unload. Look for potential hazards such as poison ivy, bees, and jagged objects like rocks or sticks, and make sure the ground is dry.

4. Set up your camp in an area where there are trees or shrubbery to protect it from high winds.

5. If you're building a fire or using a portable stove, be aware that fire is one of the main hazards in any campsite. Be sure there is plenty of water nearby in case you need to douse the flames.

6. When putting out a campfire, use a combination of dirt and water. Stir the remains and keep adding more water and dirt until the smoke is clear and the earth is cool.

7. Finally, leave the campsite as you found it. Don't leave your garbage behind. Preservation of our natural resources is something we all need to take seriously.

TOM'S TIP

I don't necessarily advocate that everyone staying in a hotel create an obstacle course in front of his door every night, but I tell this story to indicate that a hotel room is far from a bank vault when it comes to breaking and entering.

CHECKLIST FOR HOTEL SAFETY

These do's and don'ts are as applicable for domestic travelers as they are for visitors to other countries.

✔ When registering, don't give out any more information than is absolutely necessary.

✔ Once inside your room, lock the door before opening your suitcase and unpacking your valuables.

✔ Familiarize yourself with the nearest exits from the hotel in case of fire or emergency.

✔ Never "hide" things in your room and assume they'll be safe. If there's a safe in your room, use it. If not, check your valuables into the hotel safe.

✔ When you put your clothing away, arrange it in a particular manner so you'll be aware if anyone's gone through it in your absence.

✔ Check with the concierge or desk staff about which places to visit and which ones to avoid.

✔ When retiring for the night, use the deadbolt, and tip a chair against the door as an additional obstacle for would-be intruders.

✔ Never give out your room number to anyone, especially if you're traveling alone.

✔ If you're staying at a roadside motel, be sure it's well lit and that there are open passageways through which you can enter and exit.

NEAR OR FAR, PRACTICING SAFETY IS THE WAY TO STAY SAFE

Whether you're going to a local park, a shopping mall, or a foreign country, planning ahead, and practicing the Family Protection techniques with your loved ones, is the best way to ensure that you will all be able to take pleasure in your surroundings or your adventure and still be as safe as it's possible to be in a world where safety is no longer a given.

IF YOU'RE CAUGHT IN A NATURAL DISASTER

Earthquakes, hurricanes, and other natural disasters can occur anytime, in almost any place you might visit. While the odds are you won't run into one, it's still a good idea to be as prepared as possible so that you are able to stay calm, think clearly, and act rationally.

1. If the lights go out, do not light matches or cigarette lighters. Because of the gas leaks caused by many natural disasters, doing this is one of the primary causes of personal injury or death. That's why it's important to keep a working flashlight in every room. I also put a piece of glow tape on every drawer in which I store a flashlight.

2. Because many natural disasters, particularly earthquakes, cause objects to break loose and ceilings to fall, it's always wise to take cover under a heavy mattress, a sturdy table, or a desk.

3. Once you're in a secure area, stay there until the shaking or turbulence has completely stopped. Don't be tempted to run outside and see what's happening because you think it's "letting up."

4. Stay away from windows, mirrors, or anything else that might fragment. Should things start shattering, cover your eyes with something thick, or, if nothing else is available, shield your eyes with your forearm.

5. Once the activity has stopped and you have decided to leave the area, be aware that there may be a great deal of rubble or debris. Make sure you wear sturdy, skid-resistant, thick-soled shoes. Lace-up shoes are best, and you should tie them tightly to give you support and reduce the risk of ankle injury.

6. Should time permit during an emergency evacuation, take with you any medications that are essential for you or another member of your family. If possible, take important papers and any valuables that are accessible without your having to enter a dangerous area.

7. Do not use the elevators; take the stairs. If the stairwells are inaccessible, return to your safe location and wait for help.

8. Do not use land-line telephones, which, in case of damaged wiring, can cause electric shock. Never touch any exposed wires.

9. Never rush into any action; think about what you're going to do and determine whether it's the safest course before you do it.

10. Always have a preset meeting place just in case someone in your family gets separated from the group.

11. Make up an "emergency" bag and keep it in a place that will be easy to access in an emergency. In it put a battery-powered radio, flashlights with extra batteries, a first-aid kit, a few bottles of water, copies of essential documents, some cash, a spare credit card, any necessary medications, and a few clean towels. Change the materials in the bag every three months, and be sure the bag itself is waterproof.

TOM'S TIP

My goal in teaching these techniques is not to frighten anyone, but rather to provide the information and skills we all need to know so that, in any situation, we'll be prepared to act with confidence rather than to react out of fear. There's a great world out there, and the better prepared we are to navigate it safely, the more we'll be able to enjoy it.

FOUR

JUST FOR KIDS

AT A MINIATURE GOLF COURSE *with my wife and son, I noticed a group of four teenagers behind me on the course who were playing rather recklessly with the equipment. When I saw that one of them was teeing up to hit a ball in our general direction, I quickly moved my wife in front of me and placed my son between us, so that he was shielded by our bodies. Not more than a few seconds later I was hit in the lower back by a golf ball. If it had been my son rather than me, the ball would have hit him in the back of the head. This was an instance when being aware of my surroundings certainly prevented what could have been a life-altering tragedy not only for my son but for the entire family.*

AS I'VE SAID, we in Family Protection Training call children the Gift, and I believe that children are not only our most precious gift, but are also those most in need of our protection. Not just their physical size but also their open, trusting nature and natural curiosity make them vulnerable to virtually every kind of injury, purposeful or accidental, inside or outside the home. Unfortunately, however, we as parents or guardians don't always take our obligation to protect our children as seriously as we should.

This was made all too clear to me when I took a booth at a children's fair in New Jersey to promote my KNOW & GO program for teaching children about self-protection (see page 134). The day-long event attracted a variety of vendors and was well attended by parents, grandparents, and children.

After a couple of hours, I decided to conduct a little experiment. I asked the person in charge of the public address system to make an announcement that both child safety booklets and balloons were being distributed free of charge at the KNOW & GO booth in the center aisle. By the time I got back to the booth it was mobbed. My staff asked the adults if they would like a balloon, a booklet, or both. The majority of younger parents took the balloon, while the older people—generally grandparents or guardians—asked for both.

As people left with the items they had requested, I introduced myself, told them I was writing a book, and asked why they had chosen the item or items they did. Most of those who had requested only the balloon said it was to keep their child occupied, and when I asked why they hadn't also taken the booklet, they told me they didn't really believe their children were in danger because they always "kept an eye on them."

Those who took the booklet told me that they believed their children needed to be taught about safety by their parents. Some said that they lived in transitional neighborhoods and were becoming more safety-conscious as a result. One woman even looked at me with tear-filled eyes and said that she wouldn't be able to go on living if anything happened to her child.

The purpose of my self-designed experiment was to indicate how often parents focus on their children's immediate pleasure rather than on their long-term safety. Wouldn't it be just as easy and a great deal smarter to do both? If you attend an event focused on children, do take pleasure in seeing that they enjoy the outing, but at the same time make it your business to seek out the child safety booth and get whatever information is being offered. It's our job as adults to be vigilant about keeping children safe.

IT WAS AN ACCIDENT!

How often have we heard a child say, "I didn't mean it, Mommy. It was an accident!" While adults are certainly vulnerable to household injuries, children are even more so, because they are less aware of inherent dangers and are therefore less likely to take the precautions adults do to prevent them. Statistically, more children are hurt accidentally than are harmed intentionally. We adults generally approach the unknown or unfamiliar with some caution and trepidation. Children, however, are more apt to be drawn by their curiosity to anything that's "new" and therefore interesting to them, without regard for its potential danger. Since children are naturally careless, it's our job to be careful for them, first by keeping sources of danger out of sight and out of reach and then, as they grow older, by making sure they understand which common household items might actually hurt them and why. We also need to do that in a way that will educate without frightening them. We want to raise children who understand how to navigate their world without being scared to live in it.

The worst thing we adults can do to our children is to scare them into being fearful of something without explaining to them, softly but firmly, how to behave and not to behave in particular situations, and—more important—why. We talk, for example, about not touching sharp objects like knives or broken glass, but we never really explain the meaning of sharpness or how fragile young bodies really are. I realized this one day as I was watching my son make his way through the kitchen in his stocking feet when, in his haste, he accidentally knocked over a glass. It toppled to the floor, shattering into many pieces. At first he was startled, but then his curiosity took over, and even though he'd been told many times not to touch sharp objects, he decided first to yell for Mom and Dad and then to run toward us. Either he didn't associate "don't touch" with "don't step on" or he didn't make the connection between "sharp objects" and broken glass. Luckily I saw what was happening, and just as he was getting ready to take off I told him to freeze. He did what he was supposed to do, but I as a parent had failed to educate him about staying in place when something breaks, especially when he's not wearing shoes. I picked him up and carried him into the living room, and before putting him down, I checked him over thoroughly for stray shards of glass.

That incident led me to try to find out which sounds (such as breaking glass or screeching tires) were most frequently linked to intentional or unintentional childhood injuries. Having done that, I designed a program that would train children to associate particular sounds with specific responses and safe movements. The result is my international child-safety program called Tom Patire's KNOW & GO, the first-ever program that focuses on training children between the ages of four and twelve in audible recognition and the appropriate eye-hand and eye-foot reactions. Teach your children the following steps. Act them out with your children, and practice them from time to time. (You can give older children the following section to read on their own, including the guidelines for calling 911, and discuss it with them afterwards.)

KNOW & GO: WHAT KIDS SHOULD KNOW ABOUT SOUNDS AND HOW TO REACT TO THEM

I. BROKEN GLASS

KNOW: Touching or walking on broken glass can cause serious injuries, especially if you're not wearing shoes.

GO: Stop, freeze, look around to see where the broken glass is, and call for help. Do not move until help arrives!

2. CAR TIRES SCREECHING

KNOW: Drivers sometimes accidentally lose control of their vehicles because they're not paying attention or for any number of other reasons. It's no different from running into the street to chase a ball without looking to see if a car is coming.

GO: You should always look out for cars or trucks when you're playing near a street, and little kids should never try to cross a busy street without a grownup nearby. If you hear screeching tires, stop immediately, jump back away from the curb and onto the sidewalk, and run at least five steps away from where you heard the sound, then stop and look to see if the area is clear to go, or if you should stay in place. Remember, whenever you run, it should be *away* from the dangerous sound or *away* from the person you think might be dangerous.

3. PANIC-STRICKEN CROWD

KNOW: People in crowds at sporting events or in amusement parks can become aggressive when they're rushing to get in or out or, even worse, if they're spooked by something like a fire or a loud noise. When that happens, they might accidentally push you or knock you down because they don't see you and because the momentum of the crowd behind them doesn't allow them to stop even if they do see you.

GO: If this happens and you're separated from your parent, find the closest stable object to hold on to—a pillar, a railing, a seat, or a light post, for example. Wrap your arms around it and use "Sticky Hands," as described on page 95. The closer you are to whatever you're holding on to, the less chance you have of being trampled. Then yell, "Help, help, child here." Hearing the word "child" usually gets people to take notice.

To the parent: If you're with your child in this situation, pick him up and hold him close to your body, chest-to-chest, supporting his weight with one hand and protecting his neck with the other.

4. VICIOUS DOG BARKING

KNOW: Dogs often bite because they're startled by quick motions or some other type of movement that agitates them.

GO: If confronted by a barking dog, stop immediately and remain motionless. Yell for help but don't move. If the dog begins to back away, back up slowly in the opposite direction, one step at a time, pausing between steps. Don't run!

To the parent: Many parents ask what their child should do if a dog starts to attack. Running is not an option, since it would be impossible for the child to outrun the dog. If there's sand or dirt or pebbles on the spot, one option would be to train your child to pick up a fistful and throw it in the dog's eyes. If there's an unlocked car nearby, getting in it and shutting the door would be another. The best option, however, would be to teach your child to stay away from any dog that isn't on a leash, accompanied by its owner.

5. POLICE AND FIRE VEHICLES IN MOTION

KNOW: Emergency vehicles on their way to a fire or to aid someone often travel very fast, making the vehicle harder to stop and sometimes harder to control. Never run into the street, or even closer to the curb to see where these vehicles are going, because you could easily get hit.

GO: If you're playing outside and hear a fire or police siren, stop and locate the sound of the vehicle. If it's close, quickly move back at least five steps *away* from the curb and onto the sidewalk, stop, turn around, and look in all directions to see where the vehicle is coming from and where it's headed. If it's coming in your general direction, back up some more, *away* from the street.

6. SMOKE DETECTOR ALARM

KNOW: Smoke inhalation is just as dangerous as fire, if not more so. It prevents you from seeing clearly and from breathing, and it can make you panic.

GO: If you hear the smoke alarm go off, drop to the floor, crawl along the nearest wall, and yell out where you are: "Mommy, Daddy, I'm in my room, next to the wall near the dresser." Name a piece of furniture or object to help your parents to identify the wall you're next to.

7. TRAIN IN MOTION

KNOW: Train sounds echo, which means you may think they're farther away than they really are. It's always dangerous to play on or near the railway tracks.

GO: If you hear the sound of a train, stop, run a minimum of five to ten steps *away* from the tracks, then turn and look around to make sure you are clear of the tracks and a safe distance away. Look at the ground around you to make sure there aren't any rocks or ruts that might cause you to trip and fall. Then move even farther away from the tracks if you can.

8. A FRIENDLY STRANGER ASKING FOR HELP

KNOW: Never go with anyone, for any reason, whether you think you know the person or not, without your parents' permission, even if they tell you they know your parents and your parents said it was okay. People shouldn't ask a child to go anywhere with them unless the child's parent is right there to say yes.

GO: If someone asks you to help him, or offers to take you somewhere, you should immediately back up, run, and yell, "Don't touch me, stranger, stranger."

To the parent: Teach your child that if a stranger tries to snatch him, he should use "Sticky Hands" (see page 95) and hold on to a solid object, then scream to draw attention to himself. Make sure you teach your child what a "solid object" is—something like a bench, swing, or water fountain, not something that's movable. Remember, abductions happen in seconds, not minutes, so time is the key. The longer it takes to snatch the child, the greater the odds that the abduction will fail. Also note that pedophiles will play any role to convince a child to go with him. He might, for example, walk around with a dog leash and collar or even with a photograph of a dog. So work with your kids every day to impress upon them what a true stranger is.

CALLING 911

One of the most important things you can teach your child is how to call 911 and what to say to the operator:

- State your full name.
- State your complete address.
- State why you need help immediately.
- Leave the phone off the hook so that, if necessary, the call can be traced.

Our KNOW & GO child safety program is a playful yet stress-inducing course that teaches youngsters to function under pressure. The last thing they do for completion of the course is to make the 911 call when they are tired and stressed, so that their minds and bodies become familiar with what that feels like, and they will be able to perform the task in those conditions if it ever becomes necessary.

Step two of our child safety course, which we call THE LURE, teaches children how to use their environment and make themselves as much of a nuisance as possible if someone is attempting to abduct them. The third and final phase of the program is called THE AID, and teaches children what to do and how to get help in the event that something happens to a parent—if, for example, their mother falls and is unconscious or unable to get up.

These parts of the course are kept extremely confidential. Adults, other than the child's parents or guardians, are not allowed to attend. Ideally, I'd love to be able to include that information here as well, but people need to realize that Bad Guys are always trying to find out what children are being taught about self-protection. Keeping that information out of their hands is just one more thing we can do to keep our children safe.

COMMON CAUSES OF ACCIDENTAL INJURY AT HOME

Electrical outlets. Little fingers love to push little objects into holes, so be sure any outlet that doesn't have a plug in it is covered at all times. Safety covers are available at hardware stores as well as in shops selling baby equipment. Once your child is old enough, you can explain why it's important not to play with the plugs, but, to err on the side of caution, you'd be wise to leave those covers on the empty outlets.

Appliances. From large to small, appliances of all kinds pose a multitude of dangers. Obviously, stoves may be hot and refrigerator or freezer doors might slam on children's hands, but toasters, food processors, electric mixers, and electric can openers—to name just a few of the more common small appliances—might be even more dangerous. Keep these and other small appliances unplugged unless they are in use.

Household cleaning products. Virtually all such products contain poisons and must, therefore, be kept out of the reach of children until they are old enough to understand that these substances are not to be ingested. Safety locks for cabinet doors can be purchased at hardware stores and shops selling baby equipment. Additionally, it's important not to leave buckets with cleaning products or even with small amounts of water in them unattended when small children are around.

Medications. Even adults have been known to take too much of a medication inadvertently, but for children, access to both prescription and over-the-counter medications can lead to tragedy. A friend of mine once told me that her small son liked the taste of his cough medicine so much he managed to climb up on the bathroom sink and get it out of the medicine chest. Luckily he wasn't yet coordinated enough to get much of it into his mouth! Drug companies make children's medicines taste good so they'll take them. It's up to us to make sure they don't take them when they're not supposed to. And colorful pills can look a lot like candy to a child. Don't count on "childproof" caps to keep that "candy" out of the mouths of babes (and never refer to medicine as candy in front of a child).

KIDS IN THE KITCHEN

Small children love to be in the kitchen. They are fascinated with stoves, with the color of the flames, and with whatever is being cooked, not to mention the contents of cabinets and drawers. To prevent accidents, use the back burners when children are around, and always turn the pot handles away from the front of the stove. You can also purchase child safety devices to kid-proof your kitchen, like small clear plastic screens that go across the front of the stove to block a child's access to the stove and oven controls, as well as drawer and cabinet locks.

TOM'S TIP

Breakable items. As babies learn to crawl, then walk, they naturally hold on to things for balance, and sometimes breakable objects get knocked over in the process. In addition, pretty, shiny, colorful things naturally attract children's attention. If they're also breakable things, when they slip from children's hands they become shards of glass or china for children to step on or put in their mouths. Banish those objects to high places at least until children are old enough to understand that your crystal vase is not a toy to be played with. Get in the habit of not leaving glasses or breakable cups where children can reach them. Not only the container but also what it holds (hot coffee or tea, wine, or other alcoholic beverages) can be dangerous to little ones.

Sharp objects. Knives, razors, scissors, and other sharp objects are obvious dangers. Careless use on the part of adults can result in serious injury to children. Be sure to put all such objects safely away as soon as you've finished using them, and keep an eye on your children when they're in use. Remember that if they watch you use these objects, they may try to imitate your actions, so always emphasize—and demonstrate—safe usage in front of kids.

Telephone and electrical cords. Cords, even when they're not plugged in, can be dangerous. Dangling cords of all kinds get wrapped around small necks. They also offer temptation to pull, and when they're attached to heavy objects like telephones, those heavy objects can cause serious injury.

Exercise equipment. Even relatively lightweight dumbbells are heavy enough to injure a child seriously. They shouldn't be left where they might roll or be pulled off a table and land on a small head— or even a small foot. Exercise machines may look like good climbing objects, but they're high enough to cause injury in a fall. And motorized equipment should be kept unplugged when not in use.

Fire extinguishers. Fire extinguishers save lives, but they're also heavy and they contain poison. The best place to keep a fire extinguisher is in a wall bracket that's accessible to adults but out of the reach of children.

Firearms. This one should be a no-brainer. If you don't know enough to keep firearms unloaded and locked away, you really are brainless!

Garden equipment. Green hoses hidden in green lawns can be obstacles just waiting to trip up small feet. Garden tools are sharp, pointy, and dangerous. If you leave them lying around where they'll be easier for you to get to, they'll also be easier for children to get hold of and get into trouble. Pesticides, herbicides, fertilizers, and other garden chemicals should be kept entirely out of the reach of children.

KIDS AND CARS: BETTER SAFE THAN SORRY

More and more of us are spending increasing amounts of time in cars with our kids. Not only do we take road-trip vacations, but we ferry our children back and forth to school, play dates, and sports activities, and we take them with us on our rounds of errands to supermarkets, cleaners, and shops. Because we're logging all that car time, it's more important than ever for us to keep our children safe not only while we're driving, but also as they enter and exit the vehicle.

Emergency-room physicians tell terrible stories about the tragic ways children are injured in cars, one of the most common of which is what they call the "projectile effect." In the introduction to this book I recounted the story of the young woman who luckily escaped serious injury when she was hit with an empty bottle flying off the dashboard of her friend's car. Any hard object left on the dashboard, be it a baseball, a cell phone, even a purse or a wallet, becomes a potentially lethal weapon if the driver is forced to stop short. But there are other, equally dangerous and seemingly innocent ways for children to be hurt in automobiles.

CHECKLIST FOR CHILDPROOFING YOUR VEHICLE

✔ *Install and use car seats and booster seats properly.* Since there are so many of these on the market, the best thing to do if you are not sure how to install these seats is to go to the child safety officer at your local police department and ask for his expertise and assistance. He is well aware that use of child seats and booster seats is mandatory under the law and also saves lives, and he will be more than glad to help out. And once the seat is properly installed, be sure to use it every time your child is in the car, even if you're only going a few blocks.

✔ *Enter safely.* Hold the car door open with your leg to prevent it from swinging closed as your child is getting into the car while you use your hand to protect his head from hitting the doorframe.

✔ *Avoid crushed fingers.* Make sure your child keeps her hands folded in her lap until you've shut the door. It's not hard to teach even young children this simple safety habit.

✔ *Scan for potentially dangerous loose objects.* In addition to objects left on dashboards that might become dangerous projectiles, small items like pens or pencils or even plastic drinking straws left on the seat or the floor near a child have the potential to cause serious injury. Children have a tendency to poke themselves with these items even in the best of circumstances, but in a moving vehicle, a bump in the road or a sudden stop can result in a bad puncture wound or even the loss of an eye. Before you let your child in the car or before you close the door, scan the area where he will be sitting for anything that might cause this kind of injury.

✔ *Keep doors locked while driving.* Not only will this prevent a Bad Guy from getting in while you're stopped at a light or in traffic, it will also prevent the child from inadvertently opening the door while the car is in motion. Many vehicles have child safety-lock features that serve both these functions. If your car has such a feature, be sure to use it.

✔ *Keep checking on your child.* If your child is in the backseat, you can't keep turning around to make sure she's okay, but you can keep asking her questions. By soliciting a response, you'll be able to find out if she's feeling sick or has somehow hurt herself, and you'll also be bonding with your child, so use this time wisely.

✔ *Exit safely.* Whether you're pulling off the road to assist a sick or injured child or getting out because you've reached your destination, make sure that you are safely off the road and out of the way of moving traffic. Scan the area before you exit yourself, then make sure you let the child out on the side of the car opposite the flow of traffic.

✔ *Keep a first-aid kit in your car and familiarize yourself with its contents.* If you use something, be sure to replace it. If it's always in your car, you'll always have it with you.

PLAYING SAFE

Playgrounds and amusement parks are magnets for children and attractive, cost-effective venues for keeping them entertained. It's important, therefore, that we learn how to keep our children safe while taking advantage of their multiple attractions. One of the most basic tools we have for doing that is simply to remain alert and watchful. It's all too easy to let your child run off and play on the swings or the jungle gym while you "zone out." That's when children are most likely to project themselves out of the swing while it's flying high above the ground, or lose their grip on the bar when climbing to the top of a supposedly child-safe apparatus. Remember that it's your job not only to accompany your child to the playground but also to protect his safety while he's playing. Stand by, remain alert, and be ready to assist or intervene at any moment.

Not only is the equipment in playgrounds and amusement parks potentially dangerous, but other dangers might lurk there as well. Because these locations are inherently attractive to children, they are equally attractive to those who prey upon them.

I grew up in the town of Lodi, New Jersey, which was famous for the St. Joseph's feastday carnival that was held every September. It was a family tradition for my dad to take my brother, Tim, and me to the carnival because my mother's work schedule at our family's restaurant wouldn't permit her to attend. My family owned a fast-food franchise called Stewart's that was known for its famous ice-cold, homemade root beer and Texas Wieners. This particular day my father, who was a police officer in the borough of

Lodi, was called in to work on some type of emergency. Since he'd promised to take us to the carnival, he said he'd drop us off and check on us every hour just to make sure we were all right. I was ten at the time. Tim and our next-door neighbor, Mike Imparato, who was going with us, were both eleven. My father picked us up in his patrol car (this was allowed in those days) at 4:00 P.M. Before he dropped us off, he gave all three of us specific instructions to meet every hour by the zeppole stand, and for the first two hours we did just that. We met my father, he walked around with us for a while, then he gave us some money to play the games and to get refreshments, and went back to work.

At about 6:30 we were sitting by the pizza stand when an older gentleman who said he knew my father asked why we were eating pizza when we could be eating at Stewart's. My brother, who was more adventurous and outspoken than I, said, "If we had a way to get to Stewart's, we'd be eating there." The man then offered us a ride. Tim was quick to say yes, and in no time at all he'd talked Mike into going, too. "What about Dad?" I asked. "We'll have Mom call him when we get there," Tim assured me. It sounded sensible, and since I was afraid to be left alone at the carnival, I went along.

I still remember that the man drove a blue Ford pickup truck with tools in the back, as if he worked in construction. We all piled into the bed of the truck and off he drove in the direction of Stewart's. When he got there, however, he passed it right by and continued east on Route 46. He drove all the way to Teterboro Airport, which was about two miles past the restaurant, then made a U-turn and went back the other way, again passing Stewart's. Finally he turned around again, and this time when we got to the restaurant, he pulled into the parking lot and dropped us off. Before he left he helped us out of the truck, asking how we'd liked the ride. Apparently he'd wanted us to feel the wind as he drove down the highway. He figured we would like it, and Mike and Tim did, but I was the youngest and I was scared.

By that time it was 7:15 P.M., and when my mother saw us she asked where Dad was. We told her he wasn't with us and that a friend of his had brought us. Hearing that, she gave us a look that let us know we were all in trouble. She then called the Lodi police department and asked them to locate my father and tell him to come to Stewart's immediately. She was put through to the captain, who said that Dad was looking for us and had put out an all-points bulletin. When my mom got off the phone she looked over at us and said, "Your father is on his way, and you boys are in trouble." Well, she was right.

My dad was visibly upset and angry at the same time. He put us in the patrol car and took us to the police station. When we arrived, he took us into the detective bureau and asked for a certain file. Then he sat us down and asked if we knew why he was so upset. "Because we left without telling you," I said. He said yes, that's so, and you also left with someone neither he nor Mom had okayed. He opened the file and showed us a picture of a smiling boy who, he said, lived on the other side of town. He then read a missing person's report on the boy. He'd been hitchhiking to get to the St. Joseph's feast, and witnesses had seen him being picked up by an elderly man. At that point he'd already been missing for several days. By then Mike, Tim, and I all had tears in our eyes. Several days later the boy was found strangled and gagged by the Passaic River. I know that the murder investigation went on for well over six months, but I never asked my dad if they'd caught the killer. I did, however, see a police artist's sketch of him on the wall inside the department, and I remember saying to my brother that he didn't look mean.

Needless to say, I never got into a vehicle with a stranger again. The person who gave us the ride really was my father's friend, as it turned out, and he also got a lecture from my dad about giving rides to children without notifying their parents.

CHECKLIST FOR PLAYGROUND SAFETY

✔ *Be alert at all times.* You're not off duty when your child is in the playground. Rather, you ought to be on "standby alert."

✔ *Stay close by.* Not only will your child feel safer if he sees you close by, but also would-be predators will see that you are a concerned, attentive parent and will look elsewhere for their prey.

✔ *Scan for safety.* If you're in an unfamiliar playground, make sure you know where the exits are, as well as the restrooms and public telephones—you might need to find any one of these very quickly. And, if you have one, always take your cell phone. Public telephones are becoming extinct in many areas, and even when there is one, it's often out of order.

✔ *Scan for strangers.* Be alert for anyone entering the area who doesn't look as if he or she "fits in." That would include not only adults but teenagers in a playground designed for young children. If your internal alarm goes off, if you see someone who just doesn't seem to fit in, leave the area, acting casually but methodically and always with your child's safety foremost in your mind.

✔ *Stay away from strangers.* Don't get drawn into long conversations with people you don't know, and never let a stranger "play with" your child. To do that is not only to put your child in danger at the moment, it also lets him become comfortable with strangers, which could put him in danger at some time in the future. If you are drawn into talking to a stranger, particularly if the person seems in any way suspicious, withdraw from the conversation as quickly as possible and leave the area immediately. Sometimes those of us who are honest and open can be too concerned with being polite and not concerned enough about our safety and the safety of our children. We would do well to remember that in many cases the Bad Guy sees kindness as a weakness and will exploit it any way he can.

✔ *Keep your eye on the time.* Wear a watch, set a time limit, and stick to it. Children get tired when they're playing, and you get tired of watching. The more tired each of you is, the more likely you both are to be careless. Carelessness can result in accidents or worse, so it's better to leave the playground while you and your child are both alert. You can always come again another day. And it's generally best to set out for home before it begins to get dark. At dusk, it's harder for your child to see what he's doing on the swings, slide, or seesaw, and it's harder for you to see would-be predators who might be lying in wait. That's another good reason to keep your eye on the time.

As children get older, they also become more adventurous—at least until they turn into cautious adults. Do you ever look at an amusement park ride and wonder why you ever wanted to go on that thing as a child? It's because children are so fearless that we have to be extra cautious about checking out both the safety of the ride and the safety of the environment.

CHECKLIST FOR AMUSEMENT PARK SAFETY

✔ *Ask questions.* Whenever possible, find out how long the ride or attraction has been in operation. Ask when the last safety inspection took place and how often the rides are inspected. Ask if the park has experienced any recent crime-related activity. You can do this by calling the manager or security officer. The larger the venue, the easier it is to obtain this kind of information. If the person you're speaking with seems reluctant to answer your questions, let that be a warning to you.

✔ *Check out local carnivals.* Small local carnivals can be great fun for the entire family. Because they come and go, however, it might be more difficult to check them out. The best way to do that is to ask the local police. Carnivals, however peripatetic, require permits to operate, and the police are most likely the agency to have issued them. Once you're on the scene, you can also speak to the operators of the various rides; you'd be surprised at the amount and kinds of information they're willing to share.

✔ *Examine the rides.* Before allowing your child on a ride, look to see how it's set up and what's holding it together. If it makes you uneasy for any reason, try something else. Your instincts are usually correct.

✔ *Don't let them ride alone.* Once you've decided to allow a small child on a ride, one adult should always ride with him. (If it's "too scary" for you, it's definitely too scary for a little one.) If there are two of you, the second adult should wait by the exit, where the child can see him or her as he gets off the ride.

✔ *Keep them close.* When you're walking through a crowded amusement park or carnival, always keep children close. By doing that you'll be protecting them from both Bad Guys and accidental injury.

✔ *The earlier the better.* It's best to visit these venues early in the day. The later it gets, the larger the crowds, which means more potential Bad Guys as well.

PEDOPHILES AND PREDATORS:
WHAT TO TEACH YOUR KIDS

A child abducted or sexually molested—it's every parent's worst nightmare. Tragically, the two are frequently linked. Statistics published by the Federal Bureau of Investigation indicate that there is one sexual predator for every square mile in the continental United States. In addition, figures compiled by the National Center for Missing and Exploited Children say that one in every four girls and one in every seven boys will be sexually molested between infancy and the age of eighteen. In light of those frightening numbers, what can we teach our children that will reduce their risk of becoming one of those victims and increase their chances of escaping if they are ever abducted? To answer those questions, I worked with Alan J. Robinson, C.S.E., a representative of the elite Project ALERT (America's Law Enforcement Retiree Team) program of the National Center for Missing and Exploited Children. The author of "Measures to Prevent the Abduction, Kidnapping and Sexual Exploitation of Children," Mr. Robinson has trained thousands of parents, educators, police, and prosecutors in the areas of child protection and the investigation of child abductions. Below he answers some of the most frequently asked questions regarding child protection.

❝How can I educate my child about existing dangers?❞

First you have to talk to them about the kinds of dangers that do exist. Don't be shy or beat around the bush. Your child shouldn't have to guess what you're trying to say. Tell them, above all, to trust their internal alarm system. If an alarm is going off, they need to answer it by going to a trusted adult immediately.

Many victimized children identify their assailant as being "strange" or as making them feel strange. Tell your child that if someone makes him feel uncomfortable, he should trust his instincts and never hesitate to take action.

"Can children do anything to protect themselves against these criminals?"

Absolutely! Tell your child that if she senses something is wrong, she should go to the nearest pay phone and dial 911. You can dial 911 from any pay phone without putting in a coin, and in most cases you can dial from a cell phone, even one with no service. Make sure your child knows these two essential facts.

Teach your child that if he is lost or separated from you, he should go to a trustworthy adult. (Also see the section on "safety zones" in the preceding chapter. Teach your child to locate safety zones both in your town and when you are away from home.) In most cases, that would be anyone in a store who is wearing a uniform or name tag with the name of the store on it; anyone who reminds him of his grandmother; any woman pushing a stroller or holding a child's hand; any pregnant woman.

Teach your child that if she is abducted she should fight back immediately, as noisily and aggressively as possible. The harder she fights, the more likely she'll be to put her abductor in the spotlight. Since these people don't want to be caught, they'll be likely to abandon the child in order to make their getaway.

Teach your child to leave a trail. If he's being taken on foot, your child can assist law enforcement in their search efforts by leaving markers along the way. Tell him to spit on the ground. That will give search dogs a scent to pick up on. Tell him to toss aside whatever bits of clothing or personal articles he can think of; even tags or strands of hair will help the searchers to find him.

Above all, tell him to never give up and to take any opportunity he sees to escape.

TEACH YOUR CHILD HOW AND WHAT TO YELL

Most of us spend a lot of time teaching our children that it's not polite to yell or use a loud voice in public. We should also be teaching them to yell as loud as they can and what words to scream if someone is trying to kidnap or hurt them. Here are a few of the phrases that are most likely to get people's attention.

- Stranger! Stranger!
- Help! This is not my mommy [or daddy]!
- Help! This man is hurting me!

TOM'S TIP

"Should I teach my child never to talk to strangers?"

Perhaps surprisingly, the answer to that question is no. Many pedophiles and child abductors spend a great deal of time learning about the family and the life of the child they have targeted. The potential abductor may already know or have come in frequent contact with the child. Using the term "stranger" might, therefore, be confusing and lead the child to believe that only people he doesn't know can hurt him.

Remember, if child molesters looked scary, children would run away from them. Unfortunately, however, most pedophiles and child molesters appear calm and know how to use guilt to attract rather than frighten children. A pedophile might, for example, convince the child that if he doesn't help him find his puppy, it might be stolen or get hurt. Pedophiles and child molesters are, first and foremost, con men. It's better, therefore, to teach your child to handle situations than to warn him about specific categories of individuals. The child shouldn't have to decide whether any given individual might or might not be a potential Bad Guy.

If, for example, you teach your child never to get into a car, even with someone he knows, without his parents' consent, it won't matter if the individual convinces him that one of his parents has been injured or needs his help. The child will know that unless his other parent gives consent, he is not allowed in the vehicle.

If you teach your child never to get in a car, or to accept money, gifts, or drugs from anyone without first asking your permission, she won't have to think about the appropriate response, no matter who is making the offer. If a child can be confused, she can be exploited. When it comes to child safety, the simpler the logic, the easier it will be for the child to follow instructions and not be tricked.

"Is there any particular lure I should teach my child to look out for?"

Aside from offers of money, candy, or some other gift, pedophiles often lure children by asking them for assistance. Children love to think they can help a grownup. It's a fundamental desire that makes them ripe for victimization.

Teach your child that whenever an adult asks for her help, she should assist by finding her parent. Make sure she understands that it's never appropriate for an adult to ask her to keep a secret from her parents, and that if the person really wants to be helped, he or she will be happy the child has found an adult to do just that.

"What information should my child have memorized in case he is abducted or lost?"

Your child should know both parents' legal names (not just "Mommy" or "Daddy") as well as his own legal name (not just a nickname). He should know his phone number (area code included) and his full address, including the city and state.

"What can I do to keep my child safe when I'm not with him?"

As children get older, and depending on where they live, they will be out without you—riding their bikes or at the playground or athletic field. Teach them always to travel with at least one other child, even if it's to use the restroom.

Here's what one mother did when her little boy advised her that he was now "too old" to accompany her into the ladies' room. She advised her child that the only way he could use the men's room by himself was for him to sing "The Star-Spangled Banner" continuously while he was in the bathroom. She would be stationed right outside the door, and if he stopped singing for one second, she warned him, she would come marching in. It worked until the mother determined that her son was old enough to protect himself.

RESTROOM SAFETY

Any time a child—or an adult, for that matter—uses a room, such as a restroom, that is isolated and closed off, there are a few precautions to keep in mind.

- If the child is old enough to use the restroom unaccompanied, have a check-and-balance system in place. Give the child a specific time limit and wait directly outside the door. Children like to dawdle and they don't have a very good sense of time, so make sure your child understands that if he's not out in a certain amount of time, you will come in and get him. My mother always said my brother and I used to hurry because we were afraid she'd come in and embarrass us. In many cases the fear of an action is worse than the action itself.

- If the child is small, pay careful attention to anyone leaving the restroom with a child or even a bundle wrapped in a coat or a blanket. Abductors are likely to pretend the child is sick or sleeping.

- If you're an adult going to the restroom either with a child or alone, remember that the busier it is, the safer you will be. When someone is overpowered or mugged in a restroom, it's usually because he or she is alone with the Bad Guy. So, if you walk into an empty restroom, walk out and find another one that's more populated.

- Even for adults, it's safer to go to the restroom in pairs, but if you're with someone of the opposite sex, you can still establish a check-and-balance plan. Remember that the person you're with can always yell or bang on the door without actually entering the restroom.

TOM'S TIP

❝What are the most important things I can teach my child to minimize her chances of becoming a victim?❞

The two greatest tools you can give your child are self-esteem and the ability to communicate.

Teach him that he can always tell you anything! Don't overreact to whatever topic he brings up. Doing that will only make him less inclined to confide in you in the future. Boys in particular will be reluctant to tell you anything they think might result in their losing a privilege. So, for example, if your child tells you something disturbing about a friend's family member, don't tell him immediately that he can never go to that friend's house again. If and when the occasion arises, you can think of a reason to say no that's unrelated to the information he's given you.

Tell your child that her body is hers and hers alone and that no one (except a doctor, with your permission) should be allowed to touch her "bathing-suit parts." Teach her that other people's bodies are "private" too, and that she shouldn't touch their bathing-suit parts either.

❝Should I teach my child martial arts or some other self-protection technique?❞

It depends. I believe that too many self-defense and martial arts programs for children instill both their students and the students' parents with a false sense of confidence about what the child will be able to do to protect himself against a much bigger, stronger, even violent adversary.

Several years ago I saw a front-page article in the local paper about a six-year-old who had received his black belt and stating that a demonstration would be given that weekend spotlighting his talents. Since I'm a curious guy, I decided to attend. The training facility was clean and nicely decorated. On the walls hung many pictures of children in brown belts and black belts. The demonstration was entertaining, the instructor was good, and the kids were better than average. As a finale, the little—and I do mean little—six-year-old came out and did a martial arts form. Following that, he took on four guys, each six feet tall or better, who were attacking in a group, by using self-defense moves. The self-defense was comical at best, but all the people in the audience were commenting on how cute the kid was and how well he'd be able to protect himself on the street.

At the end of the demonstration, the head instructor talked about how many six- and seven-year-olds in his school would soon be black belts, and explained that they had a special program specifically to train these children to become black belts at a early age. I admit that it was a good business ploy, but I believe that ultimately it will be harmful for kids that young to really believe they can beat up people who are a lot bigger and stronger than they are.

I do, on the other hand, believe that martial arts training can be good for kids, so long as the program doesn't center only on fighting skills. Teaching kids to be more attentive in school, to respect others, to be better human beings, to be safety conscious, and to have confidence in themselves is what I feel the martial arts are really about.

A child might get lucky and be able to take down a Bad Guy, but to me it's more important that his mind be trained to react calmly and confidently under pressure. Remember that fear overrides other emotions and leads the body to doubt itself. If we as adults fall prey to this kind of doubt, what makes us think our children won't? My approach has always been to teach kids a well-rounded program that stresses awareness and teaches how to outsmart the Bad Guy, not how to beat him up.

So if it's a question of teaching martial arts over teaching safety and awareness, the intelligent decision would be safety first and foremost.

WHAT YOU CAN DO TO MAKE YOUR CHILD SAFER

In addition to the Family Protection Training techniques we've already discussed, there are things you can do before, during, and after your child is either lost or abducted to help ensure his ultimate safe return. Prevention always comes first, but must be reinforced with thorough preparation.

Be Prepared for the Worst and Hope It Never Happens

I pray as much as you do that you never have to experience the pain of having your child go missing. If the worst should happen, however, being prepared in advance can vastly improve the chances that he'll be found quickly. According to the National Center for Missing and Exploited Children, almost 75 percent of abducted children who become victims of homicide are killed within the first two or three hours of being taken. The faster you can provide law-enforcement officials with essential information, the more likely it is that your child will be found alive.

A recent poll of parents conducted by the center in a non-stressful interview environment determined that 34 percent didn't know their child's eye color, height, or weight. If that's true, the increased stress of knowing your child is missing would make it even more difficult to recall this information. That's why it's so important to keep an updated record on hand, preferably on your person (in your purse or in your wallet) to give the police immediately.

CHECKLIST FOR CHILD IDENTIFICATION

✔ In your wallet or purse, keep a typed record of your child's identifying characteristics. These should include full name, date of birth, social security number, height, weight, eye color, hair color, skin tone, and birthmarks or other uniquely identifying characteristics. An up-to-date photo showing your child in a normal, natural pose should be kept with this record. Be sure the information as well as the photograph is updated regularly. Children grow quickly, almost month to month at some stages, and you don't want to be guessing how much they've grown or how much weight they've gained when you're trying to describe them accurately in an emergency situation.

✔ Other useful identifying features would include braces or glasses, body piercings, nicknames, favorite and least favorite foods, any medications he must take (such as insulin for diabetes or an inhalant for asthma), and the name of a pet or favorite toy.

✔ Make sure that you or your dentist has up-to-date records. Dental records can be essential for identification. If you're not sure whether your dentist's records are accurate, or if you know he isn't reachable on a twenty-four-hour basis, you can make an impression of your child's mouth on your own. To do this, cut a clean, flat section about three inches square from a Styrofoam container (such as the ones you get hamburgers in at a fast-food restaurant). Tell your child to bite into the middle of the Styrofoam using all his teeth. Then write the child's name on the Styrofoam. It's important to update this record every few months to ensure its accuracy, particularly if your child is wearing braces or has missing teeth.

✔ Keeping fingerprint cards and DNA samples may sound extreme, but if your child is ever missing, I can assure you that these things won't seem extreme anymore. Many law-enforcement agencies will do the fingerprinting for you. Call your local police precinct and ask if they will oblige. You can make it seem like fun for your child, and it's best to have this done professionally. Your pediatrician can take a DNA sample and show you the best way to store it. Properly stored, such samples will keep for many years.

✔ Train yourself to notice exactly what your child is wearing every time she leaves the house. This should include the color, style, and fabric of everything from shirt to socks and shoes. Paying attention to these details will help to identify your child more quickly and perhaps save her life.

✔ Remember that the abductor may modify some of your child's identifying characteristics, such as hair color, clothing, and eyeglasses, which is why it's so important to keep accurate records of those charac-

SAFEGUARDING YOUR CHILD'S NAME AND ADDRESS

My son attends a very progressive school, and his kindergarten teacher, Debbie Welch, is not only attentive to the kids but also highly safety-conscious. She teaches the children to keep their names and addresses out of sight, inside rather than outside their notebooks and backpacks, for example. When I asked my son if he understood why Mrs. Welch does this, he told me it was "so that strangers don't know our names and where we live." I commend Mrs. Welch because she is making safety part of the educational process.

If you remember what I've already said about pedophiles being con men, you'll realize that giving them access to your child's full name and address will make their job that much easier.

TOM'S TIP

teristics that can't be changed—weight and height, birthmarks, scars, or other uniquely identifying physical abnormalities. Since, by the way, shoes are harder to change than clothes, an abductor will often neglect to change the victim's shoes—a good point for parents to remember.

CHECKLIST FOR DESCRIBING AN ABDUCTOR

✔ *Description of person.* Height, weight, eye color, hair color and style, clothing, distinguishing features such as eyeglasses, scars, baldness.

✔ *Description of vehicle,* including color, license plate number, state, and direction in which the car was traveling.

✔ If you saw the person coming out of a store, tell the authorities. He might have charged a purchase on a credit card or been captured on a video surveillance camera.

KEEPING YOUR CHILD SAFE AT SCHOOL

Since my son started attending school, I've taken it upon myself to make schools safer for children. Here are some suggestions you can give to school officials to make your child's school a safer place.

- Make sure all outside doors are closed and locked during school hours. Most schools have a buzzer system that allows visitors to identify themselves through an intercom and get buzzed in. Higher-tech systems consist of a small covert camera by the door with a monitor in the office that allows the person inside to see who is being buzzed in. This system is cost-effective and makes the school a safer haven for our children.

- Make sure that all classroom doors are kept closed during class so that the teacher will be more aware of someone walking into her class.

- Implement a customized ID and pass program, in which staff and students have identification cards with a photo and the school logo. Guests would sign in and receive a pass, which they would have to wear on the premises and return when they left. Institute a system for keeping track of these passes so that they don't fall into the wrong hands.

- Make sure the halls are monitored either by teachers or a staff specially trained for that purpose.

- Make sure all children and school personnel are trained in how to make a 911 call.

- Develop and implement a plan of action for dealing with strangers inside the school or on the school premises.

- Train designated, responsible school personnel to act as a response team in case of a violent encounter or an abduction.

TOM'S TIP

BE ALERT TO SIGNS OF DANGER

Being alert can save not only your own child but someone else's child as well. Children do get angry and scream hateful things at their parents. It's not unusual for a child who's upset or angry to yell "I hate you!" at his mother or father. But if you ever hear a child screaming "That's not my daddy," it's almost certain he's being abducted. Contact the authorities at once, and provide as much descriptive information as you can.

TOM'S TIP

WHEN YOU DISCOVER YOUR CHILD IS MISSING

You're walking through a mall or shopping in a supermarket and you're sure your child is right next to you. But then you turn around and she's gone. Instantly your adrenaline surges and you go into panic mode. If you haven't internalized what it is you should do, you'll probably be frozen in fear just long enough for an abductor to get away. Memorize the "three S's" to help ensure your child's safety:

1. **SCAN** the immediate area from left to right, which, as we've discussed, is the natural way for your eyes to move and the best way to process information about your surroundings.

2. **SHOUT** your child's name (crouch down, as discussed, to take your child's height and hearing into account), and if he doesn't appear at once,

3. **SCREAM** as loud as you can to draw attention to yourself and the situation. Just as teaching your child to struggle and scream will help him to draw attention to himself and perhaps scare the abductor into letting him go, your screaming might just induce the kidnapper to drop your child and run for his life.

If you do scan, shout, and scream and your child suddenly reappears because she's been playing hide-and-seek, use the opportunity to reinforce her understanding of why that behavior is so danger-ous. Tell your child how much you love her and how worried you were when you couldn't find her. Explain again why leaving your side in a public place can be dangerous. And do understand that no decent, rational human being will criticize you or hold you ac-countable if you should become emotionally upset because you thought your child had been abducted.

LOOKING FOR WOLVES IN SHEEP'S CLOTHING

If you're sending your child to day care, enrolling him in a day camp, or sending her to a play group, or if your child asks to join a club or some other type of organization, you can't be too careful about checking the credentials of those who will be in charge of his safety. These people are acting *in loco parentis* and should expect to have their backgrounds scrutinized. Don't be afraid to ask ques-tions or to check references. Any irregularity, such as a gap in the person's employment record or dates of employment that don't ap-pear to be accurate, should trigger warning signals. Refusal or re-luctance to provide the information you seek should set off your internal alarm system as well. If your instinct tells you something's not quite right, don't put your child in that person's care.

DIGITAL DANGER: PREDATORS ON THE INTERNET

Thanks mainly to the media, most parents are now alert to the dan-gers their children—particularly adolescents and teenagers—might encounter on the Internet. It is nevertheless worth repeating that it's not merely a matter of trusting your children not to log on to inap-propriate websites or enter the wrong chat rooms. Rather, it's even more important that your children understand the access anonymity can provide those who wish to do them harm. Your child may think it's fun to give false information about him- or herself; but if he or she can do it, so can the person at the other end of the "conver-sation."

WHEN YOU'RE HIRING A SITTER OR A NANNY

One of the biggest concerns many of my clients—as well as my wife and I—have is how to find an honest and responsible person to care for their child. According to the FBI's National Incident-Based Reporting System (NIBRS), baby-sitters are responsible for 4.2 percent of all reported crimes against children.

These are the steps I follow when I'm doing a background check on a potential baby-sitter or private tutor. If you are hiring one through a service, ask the agency to provide the background information listed below. If you are doing this privately, a reputable private investigations firm will do the checking for you. Expense should not be your main concern when you're trying to find the right person to take care of your most valuable possession—your child!

1. *Criminal history check.* Do this on both the state and federal level.

2. *Sexual offender check.* (Different states have different laws that affect the privacy of sexual offenders, and some states are much stricter than others.) Unlike certain other types of crimes, sexual offenses are kept on record by law-enforcement agencies beyond seven years and are tracked by agencies such as the FBI from one jurisdiction to another.

3. *Motor vehicle driving history.* This will indicate whether the person is responsible behind the wheel and will turn up any speeding tickets as well as offenses such as DUI and reckless driving.

4. *Current and previous addresses.* Frequent changes of address might indicate a pattern of instability and should raise a red flag for further investigation.

5. *Professional license certification and verification.* If the person claims to be licensed or certified to do a particular job, call the organization to see if his certification is valid and what it actually certifies him to do.

6. *Reference verification.* Always ask for references and check them thoroughly. Ask the previous employer the following questions:

- How long did she work for you?

- How was she with the kids?

- What was your relationship with this person?

- Was she ever late?
- Do you consider her trustworthy?
- Did you ever notice her smoking or drinking around the children?
- How is her temperament with the kids?
- Is this just a job for her, or does she really enjoy her work?
- What types of activities did she do with the kids?

7. *Personal certifications.* Find out if she is certified in adult/infant CPR, fire safety, and basic first aid for adults and children. Then ask her to show you her current certification card.

8. *Meeting at a neutral location.* Make your first meeting with a baby-sitter at a restaurant or diner so that if anything seems "not right" to you, you can politely say "no thank you" and the person won't know where you live. If the first meeting goes well, you can arrange a second meeting at your residence.

TOM'S TIP

Direct adult supervision is the best way to protect your child from digital danger as well as any other kind. Realistically, however, you can't be watching over his or her shoulder the entire time he's online. And, very often, as parents, we're so grateful for the respite that comes from knowing our child is at home, quiet, busy, and at least theoretically safe, that we might be less vigilant than we should. We can, nevertheless, establish a few simple rules for both ourselves and our children that will mitigate the chances of their becoming the targets of Internet crime.

CHECKLIST FOR INTERNET SAFETY

✔ Keep the computer in a central location such as the kitchen or the family room, rather than in your child's bedroom. That way he won't be isolated for hours at a time, and you can glance over once in a while to see what's on the screen even while you're engaged in other matters.

✔ Take an interest in how your child is spending her time online. Ask what she's learning. Your show of involvement might encourage her to talk openly without your invading her privacy.

✔ Consider using a pseudonym for your child or not listing his name, depending on what your Internet service provider will allow.

✔ Don't give out your own identifying information in any chat room or on any public Internet bulletin board. You might just be inviting a Bad Guy into your home.

✔ Make sure your child completely understands how dangerous it is to meet anyone in the flesh whom he's known only through "virtual" contact. Emphasize how truly anonymous Internet contact really is.

✔ If you should become aware of any transmission or viewing of child pornography while you're online, report it immediately to the National Center for Missing and Exploited Children by calling 1-800-843-5678.

IN SUMMARY

Your child is your most precious gift, and it's your job—your loving obligation—to keep him or her safe from both accidental injury and deliberate victimization by doing the thinking and planning a child can't do. Happily, our children are generally oblivious to the dangers they might find both at home and in the outside world. That's as it should be. We adults, however, need to educate them, at the appropriate time and in words that won't frighten them, about what they can do to keep themselves safe. And we need to take responsibility for protecting them in whatever ways we can.

FIVE

WHY PEOPLE DO BAD THINGS— AND WHAT YOU CAN DO ABOUT IT

A FRIEND OF MINE *from New Jersey had decided to take his wife to see a Broadway play. Knowing how difficult (and expensive) it is to park in midtown Manhattan, and not wanting to drive in the city, he decided it would be best if they parked in Hoboken and took the PATH train across the river.*

On the train, he and his wife ate the sandwiches they'd bought at a local delicatessen and, because they were unfamiliar with subways, were treating their ride more like entertainment than a trip on public transportation. In fact, they were so busy not paying attention that they missed their stop. When they did finally get off, they were in unfamiliar territory, and like most people who are lost, they began to wander aimlessly, hoping to figure out which way to go. When they didn't seem to be getting anywhere, the husband decided to ask directions from a man he saw standing outside a store, holding a newspaper. "You can go a couple of ways," he said, "but let me show you a shortcut." And with that he walked them around a corner to an alley that cut between two buildings. "Why go this way?" my friend's wife asked. "Why not?" said the man, pulling out a knife that had been hidden in the newspaper. Holding the knife to my friend's wife's throat, he warned the man not to make a sound or he'd cut his wife's throat, and then directed him to empty his pockets. The husband did as he was told, and the mugger then pulled off the woman's gold necklace and told the couple to sit down with their backs to the wall and count to a hun-

dred before they moved. Again they followed directions, and they got away with their lives if not with their valuables. But they have never returned to the city, and it's now been four years since the incident occurred.

NO MATTER HOW vigilant you are, there's always a chance that you will, at some point in your life, be unable to avoid a violent or potentially violent confrontation. If and when that happens, no matter how much martial arts training you may have had in a safe, controlled environment, it will be your mental rather than your physical training that will make the difference between escaping unharmed and becoming a victim.

Mental training involves not only developing a firm belief in your own abilities, but also learning to "read the mind" of your potential attacker. Criminals, unfortunately, don't follow the rules of civilized, legal combat. They don't "play fair," and that makes it difficult for law-abiding citizens who do. Most of us have been brought up to believe that, ultimately, good will triumph over evil, and I believe that, too. I also know, however, that along the way the good guys will lose a few battles and innocent lives will be lost.

If you're lucky, the closest you've come to a violent encounter is in the movies or watching *Law & Order* in the comfort of your own home, and that's great. The problem is that even though on some level you know better, you still want to believe that the way crime is depicted in the media is true. Not only that, but the cops and the prosecutors who appear on those programs always come back to fight another week while the criminals go to prison. Not long ago, my wife and I were discussing a news segment we'd seen about a police officer who'd lost his life in a shootout when my son, having overheard our conversation, turned to me and said, "Daddy, don't be sad. He'll be back on TV next week." His sweet innocence reminded me that, as a child, I too had that kind of innocence. I never doubted that my father, who was a police officer, would return home safely every day. Since then, however, hard experience has taught me how naïve my faith really was.

Although some might protest that innocence is bliss, I believe that a realistic understanding of the criminal mind, and realistic preparation for unforeseen events, is the best defense we have against the Bad Guys out there who wish to harm us.

A LOOK AT THE MIND OF VIOLENCE

I'm sure that each one of you has some preconceived notion about what goes on in the mind of a violent criminal. In fact, however, those who perpetrate violence think as differently from one another, and for as many different reasons, as the rest of us. Getting a "read" on the way different kinds of people think can let you know how best to respond, which will, in turn, vastly increase the odds of your walking away unharmed. Understand that the mindset of a Bad Guest is drastically different from that of a Bad Guy. The key is to identify correctly both the situation and the type of person with whom you are dealing.

The Chemically Unbalanced

The chemically unbalanced or drug-altered mind goes through a wide range of quickly shifting emotions and is beyond rational thought. The person who is high on drugs—particularly amphetamines or "speed"—and who gets involved with a criminal act is very often nervous and extremely unpredictable because his heart is racing, causing both his mind and his body to run on fast-forward. Should he be armed, particularly with a handgun, his nervousness or agitation might lead to his unintentionally discharging his weapon. When that happens, the perpetrator is likely to go through a litany of mixed emotions.

If the perpetrator's intended victim is properly trained and prepared, however, his chances of survival are very good because the person with a chemically unbalanced mind is unable to think clearly and decisively. His indecisiveness means that he will be less able to act quickly and he will be concentrating more on his thought processes than on his actions. That indecision provides a window of opportunity for a quick-thinking, fast-acting, properly trained person.

The Mentally Deranged

When you're confronted by someone who is mentally unbalanced, you'd be wise always to expect the unexpected, and to act as quickly as you can to defuse the situation once his intentions become apparent. I had the dubious privilege of witnessing this kind of mind in action when I was doing masonry work to help pay my way through college. One day, one of the men in our group asked the foreman when he would be paid, and was told that everyone got paid on Friday. The worker said he wanted to be paid immediately. The foreman repeated that everyone got paid on Friday, that the next day was Friday, and that he'd be paid then along with everyone else. The worker turned and walked away, got a drink of water, and picked up his shovel as if he were about to go back to work. Instead, however, he swung the shovel at the foreman's head. He was quickly restrained, but the most bizarre aspect of this bizarre scene was that he never said a word, either during the attempted assault or when he was restrained. His eyes were so blank that it was obvious he had completely lost touch with reality. Later I learned from my father that the man was, at the time, on a work-release program from a mental institution because the authorities were testing him to see how he would "fit into society." I guess they got their answer that day.

Sometimes when the mind is so impaired, it appears that the body is able to summon a kind of superhuman strength. When confronted by a person who is mentally impaired, your best chance for survival is to act quickly to disrupt your would-be attacker's motor abilities before he is able to strike. As I teach my students in our CDT (Compliance, Direction, Takedown) courses, if you can't "get" your assailant, he will "get" you. In chapter six I'll be providing you with a few simple techniques—five easy-to-do moves—that will level the playing field in cases where you need to act fast and brain must triumph over brawn.

The Wannabe

The wannabe's mindset is a lot like that of the playground bully, and is more frequently found in a Bad Guest than in a Bad Guy. The wannabe puts up a tough front and preys on the weak because of his own insecurities. To feed his own ego, he becomes aggressive and confrontational toward those whom he perceives as passive or meek. If he sees that a victim isn't standing up to him, the wannabe will do whatever he can to terrorize him, and possibly harm him physically as well. Very often, however, when someone does stand up to this kind of person and speaks calmly in a confident voice, he will back off and back down. The wannabe, in other words, knows how to talk the talk but he very often can't walk the walk.

I saw this in a real-world situation when several of us were working a protection detail in California. We were waiting outside a building for the motorcade carrying our client to pull up. Next to us, I noticed a bus stop where a slightly built gentleman of Asian descent was sitting on a bench holding a newspaper, apparently waiting for his bus. Because the bench was broken, there was room for only one person. Just a few minutes later a large man approached the bus stop and loudly demanded that the seated man get up. The Asian man just looked at him and did not say a word. The other man, who was more than six feet tall, then bent over and yelled at him to get up because he wanted to sit. Again no reply. Finally he threatened the Asian man, screaming, "If you don't get up right now, I will rip you out of that seat." Hearing this, the Asian gentleman said, "Sir, if you put your hands on me, I will have no choice but to defend myself." He then stood up, put down his newspaper, stepped back, and raised his hands, assuming a stance that was somewhere between that of a boxer and that of a martial artist. He looked the aggressor right in the eyes and said, "There will be no more talking." The other man stared at him for about thirty seconds and then, as quickly as he'd come, he walked away, leaving the Asian man to his newspaper and his seat.

Later that week I saw the Asian gentlemen in a delicatessen where I was ordering sandwiches for my team. I told him that I admired the way he'd handled himself at the bus stop, and when he looked at me quizzically, I explained that I'd been with a group of men outside the adjacent building, and that we'd been on a protection assignment. "If my first responsibility hadn't been to my client," I said, "I'd have given you a hand, but from the looks of things it seemed that you didn't need my help."

He smiled then, and I asked where he'd received his martial arts training. "To be very honest, sir," he said, "I have none."

"But you stood up to that guy," I said, surprised. "You even took a stance."

"Yes," he said. "Many years ago as a kid, growing up in Korea, I had some training at the educational facility I attended. But knowing I was not going to give up my seat, and realizing that true warriors do not have big mouths, I took the challenge because I believed he would back down. I am small," he went on, "but Asian people are associated with the martial arts. So I used what I had going for me, and it worked."

I shook his hand and said, "Well, I bought it."

"So did the other guy," he replied.

The Seasoned Mind

The person with a seasoned mind has no need to "prove himself" to anyone, but will do what he has to in any given situation. His common sense and self-preservation skills have been tested over time, which means that your actions or the circumstances of the situation will most likely determine whether he attacks, defends himself, or retreats. His is the mindset I try to instill in the good guys through Training for Life. We need more "seasoned" people in this world who are law-abiding, who have nothing to prove, but who are prepared to deal with an unexpected or violent situation in a way that is both legal and physically appropriate.

Just a few months after 9/11, I'd been speaking at a bodyguard convention in Las Vegas and decided to take a red-eye flight back to New Jersey to be with my family. When I arrived at the airport there was a long line of people waiting to go through security. Tempers flared, as they do in any crowded airport when people are in a rush to get home, and in this case the situation was exacerbated by the fact that many were still dealing with the aftereffects of having had a wild time in Vegas.

Then, all of a sudden, a man rushed the line, saying he was late for his flight. In his haste, he knocked over an elderly lady who was being accompanied by her middle-aged son. People started yelling at the man, who, instead of stopping to apologize, yelled back and continued on his dash.

I helped the woman's son get his mother to her feet, and then went to fetch her a glass of water. We finally got through security and I sat with them as we waited for our flights to be called. As luck would have it, the man who had rushed the gate must have had the wrong flight information, because he was waiting at the gate with us.

As we all sat there, he began to stare at the man and his mother, and then to verbally abuse them. At first the woman's son remained quietly attentive to the situation, but when the stranger got out of his seat and came over to where we were sitting, he stood up, looked the aggressive Bad Guest directly in the eye, and stared. Meanwhile, I took the elderly woman by the arm and led her to the seats behind us that were out of harm's way.

The Bad Guest again took up his verbal tirade, and that's when the woman's son looked at him and said, calmly but firmly, "In your haste you knocked over my elderly mother, and, like any good son, I try to protect my parents. So, although I'm not here to be violent, I will do whatever I have to in order to protect the people I love." The troublemaker just looked at him as the son stared back expressionlessly and said, in a sharp, clear voice, "Apologize to my mother and we are done with this."

The offender's entire demeanor changed in an instant. First he apologized to the son. Then he walked over to the mother and apologized to her. When he left, the son sat down next to us and thanked me for looking after his mother. The mother smiled and kissed her son, then turned and thanked me.

We parted ways, and as I sat on my plane I said to myself, "Man, that guy was the whole package—calm, cool, a family protector, and confident of his self-preservation skills." He was, in fact, the perfect example of a seasoned, law-abiding individual. Had he been a criminal with the same seasoned mind, he would have made a formidable adversary.

The Serious Person

The serious person is a thorough professional who fits into society on a daily basis but can become a deadly adversary whenever he chooses. He's trained himself to the peak of physical perfection and has developed such a totally positive mindset that he cannot be intimidated, no matter the circumstances. He is completely unemotional and deals with the moment without any self-doubt or self-recrimination. People with this kind of mind are the ninjas of the world—highly trained bodyguards or professional assassins, members of the military special forces or master criminals. You won't encounter them holding up supermarkets or mugging victims in the streets, and unless you have the misfortune to get in their way or to be in the wrong place at the wrong time, you probably have no reason to fear them.

Being in the wrong place at the wrong time is, however, exactly what happened when I was providing security for a manufacturing mogul who had gone to Santo Domingo to investigate the possibilities for setting up factories in the Dominican Republic. The client wanted to eat at one of the better Spanish restaurants in town, so we made a reservation for seven o'clock and took a table near the rear exit—just in case—with me facing the main entrance.

It was about ten past eight when a gunshot rang through the window and everyone in the restaurant hit the floor. In the midst of the chaos, I kicked open the back door and pulled the client out with the help of a colleague. I then instructed my colleague to stay with the client as I got the car and backed it up to the exit. We threw the client in back and took off while the mayhem was still going on.

Once we were safely back at our hotel, I called the local police, and an officer came over to speak with us. He told us that a local businessman had been assassinated and that our client was not the target. The assassin had walked onto the veranda surrounding the restaurant and fired a single bullet into the head of the business-man, who had been seated no more than a foot from the window, having dinner by himself. The shooting had all the earmarks of a professional hit. No traces of the killer were left, and no identifica-tion was made.

The Extreme Mindset

People with an extreme mindset are the ones who bring fear and chaos into our lives. They embrace death and have no compassion for others because they have no compassion for themselves. To make the rest of us understand how "serious" they are, they will perform irrational and shocking acts like slashing a person's throat or shooting a hostage in the head while a witness looks on. They are the fanatics, the suicide bombers, the religious cult followers whose twisted "morality" is beyond the comprehension of any rational thinker. But make no mistake, they are soldiers in an army that tar-gets areas for mass destruction and mass casualties, and whether or not we believe in their cause, we must understand that they will not hesitate to take a life, or even hundreds of lives, if they can.

The proof of their dedication and intent is the tragedy of Sep-tember 11, 2001. The terrorists' methodically planned mission not only left an unprecedented number of casualties in its wake, it also disrupted thousands of businesses, affected the world economy, changed air travel as we had always known it in the United States, and forever influenced our own lives and the lives of those who will come after us.

If any good is to come from that horror, it will be our heightened awareness that acts of violence can and do occur when we least expect them, and that we need to learn whatever we can about protecting both ourselves and our loved ones. The more people realize that they must take responsibility for educating themselves about personal protection, the more good people will have a chance to survive against extremists. Without training and without belief in your ability to survive, you will be leaving your fate in the hands of those who place no value on either your life or their own.

MOST OF US are unlikely to come in contact with a "serious" criminal, and while we all know that there are many extremists all over the world, our chances of falling victim to one of their acts is statistically extremely unlikely. Those whom we most need to understand and protect ourselves against are the chemically unbalanced, the deranged, the wannabe, and the seasoned professional, any one of whom might unexpectedly cross our path in the course of daily life.

THE ANATOMY OF AN ALTERCATION

How an altercation will unfold, or even if one will occur in any particular situation, depends on the minds and personalities of the people involved, as well as on the nature of the situation. Some people go through life "just itching for a fight." It almost seems as if they're daring us to challenge them so that they can show us how tough they are—or how tough they think they are. Put two of those people together, and trouble is bound to ensue. At the other end of the spectrum are those who hate confrontation and will do almost anything to avoid it. Challenge them and they'll walk away if they can; just take it, if they can't; or simply fall apart and beg for mercy. The survivor is usually the person who knows when to defend himself, when to walk away, and when to make a preemptive strike. Knowing how to read another person's body language and expression is one of the best tools we can have for making that kind of decision.

As a protection professional, I have been involved with so many different types of personalities that I am quickly able to judge who will be violent and who may just be posturing. In fact, however, all of us ought to know how to recognize all types of personalities, which is why I've devised the following list of characteristics to look for.

Confrontational Styles

- *The Pacifist* will take any kind of abuse and do anything to avoid or end a confrontation. His first choice would be to walk away, but, if necessary, he'll beg for mercy rather than doing anything to defend himself. These people represent the majority of the population in today's society. They are easy to spot because they will do just about anything to avoid an argument, including admitting they're wrong even when they're right.

- *The Agitator* will stage a relentless verbal assault even though his physical skills may be mediocre at best. Like the bully, he seeks to dominate through verbal intimidation. And, like the bully, he loves to show off in front of other people and become the center of attention. These people are antagonistic blowhards who need to bolster their own shallow egos by denigrating others.

- *The Confronter* looks forward to taking on anyone and everyone who crosses his path for no particular reason and without any encouragement. He will go out of his way to look for trouble, and will use any excuse to get into a fight that will very quickly become violent. He's the guy who will go out of his way to bump into you in passing rather than get out of your way. He is generally a truly unhappy individual who feels that the world has treated him unjustly. He may have a history of violence and very often was abused as a child.

- *The Equalizer* is the person who takes the initiative. He listens and will try to defuse the situation if he can, but he's also prepared to act. He's well trained and confident both mentally and physically, and if his buttons are pushed, he can be a potential aggressor's worst nightmare. Spotting this person usually isn't hard. He is the non-aggressor, the one who's calm in the midst of a storm. Whatever may be going on around him, he keeps his composure and acts in accordance with whatever the situation demands.

BODY LANGUAGE AND WHAT IT HAS TO TELL US

Just like French or Italian, "body language" is something we can learn to read and speak, if and when we decide to become students of human nature. Learning to read another person's body language may take some work, but doing so can help us to tell the difference between people who are "safe" and those who might be trouble waiting to happen. And if we can learn to control our own body language, we can speak silently to others in a way that lets them know we're alert, prepared, and not to be messed with.

I devised a little experiment of my own to prove my own theories about what other people read from and how they react to the body language of others. I'd been asked to address an American Society of Industrial Security convention in San Antonio, Texas. I took an inexpensive flight and wore soft colors and a comfortable, cozy-looking shirt. I was purposely projecting a friendly image. On the flight, I made eye contact and smiled at my fellow passengers. By the time we landed, I'd made more than twenty new acquaintances, all of whom wished me the best and said they hoped to see me on the return flight.

On the flight home, I wore dark colors and spoke to no one. When people looked at me, I glared into their eyes until they turned away. I saw three people on the plane whom I'd met on the flight out, but when they looked at me I gave them an expressionless stare. I could tell they had absolutely no idea I was the same guy they'd met just a few days before. When we landed, my fellow passengers made it a point to allow me to deplane ahead of them.

I'd certainly proved my own point, which is that body language has its own distinct vocabulary that "speaks" to others in a loud, clear voice. Understanding that language is simply a matter of learning the vocabulary and being alert to what it's saying. We speak with our eyes, with our walk, even with our posture when seated. Knowing where to look and what to look for, as well as how to do the looking, is a key part of training the body and mind to work together for our protection.

Reading What the Eyes Are Saying

In my world, the saying "the eyes are windows to the soul" couldn't be more true. Here is a checklist I developed to help you determine what another person's eyes are telling you about his soul.

- *Insecure eyes* will meet yours for only a second before they turn down and away and never look back. Bad Guys often target people with this look because insecure eyes project a lack of self-confidence.

- *Glaring eyes* look you up and down with a cocky, overconfident stare. They are likely to be the sign of a person who will provoke rather than defuse a potentially volatile situation.

- *Dead eyes* look right through you as the person talks. They may be a sign that "the lights are on but no one's at home," and they should let you know that this is a home you don't want to enter.

- *Crazy eyes* might be darting all about. They tell you right away that the person is unstable and therefore completely unpredictable. He may act impulsively or for reasons governed by a totally irrational thought process.

- *Trained eyes* look at you and scan the surrounding area at the same time. These are the eyes of a seasoned, experienced professional whose confidence is backed by realistic training. Very few people have these trained eyes, but those who do are the ones who inspired the saying "He can kill you with his eyes."

TRAINING YOUR EYES

Your eyes relay messages to other people. By using your mind, you can train your eyes to send the messages you want. Years ago I had a student named Steve who, when he began training with me, did not even have the confidence to look you in the eye. As he started to believe more and more in himself and what he was learning, however, not only did he develop the confidence he needed to look directly into the eyes of those he was talking with, but his entire personality changed as well. Even his wife told me that she had never seen such a change in a person. "He takes me dancing now and even goes shopping with me," she said.

The key to Steve's success was that, as a result of his training, he had found his comfort zone. The look in his eyes reflected his new image of himself. He was confident now, rather than afraid.

In many cases, self-confidence leads to assertiveness. When I first realized the eyes were essential to the image one projects, I began to train myself not only to read the eyes of others but also to project the "look" I wanted others to see. I did this by going alone to various shopping malls at different times of day, when they were more or less crowded.

To perfect what I call the Glance, I chose a store with which I wasn't familiar and located it on the mall map. Then I started walking toward my destination looking straight ahead and glancing to my left and right every fifteen feet or so, letting my subconscious mind process the information. By doing this you can train yourself to see more and more while looking for it less and less.

The Passive Glare comes in handy when you think the wrong people are focusing on you. To develop the Glare, again you can use the mall as your training ground. This time, walk against the flow of traffic so that you can see everyone in your path. As you walk toward them, should they not move aside, wait until the last minute to give them the right of way, keeping your eyes focused on theirs and projecting a sense of urgency. You should be walking at a fair pace without running or appearing to be hurrying. Keep your chin up and your eyes wide open. Focus not only on the person in front of you but on whatever is in your direct line of sight. If you do this correctly, people will read the sense of urgency in your eyes and will clear the way for you.

The Stare is the look to use when you think someone is targeting you or a member of your family. To perfect it, go to a food court in a mall and get something to drink—not something to eat. The reason for this is that many people look around while they're enjoying a beverage. Find a seat at or near the center of the food court and, while you're drinking, look around in a non-offensive manner. Try to focus on someone who is staring at you. And, yes, people do stare. When you find that person, make eye contact and look directly into his eyes for a few seconds. Then sip your drink while maintaining eye contact. Hold that look for ten seconds and then look away. Wait another ten seconds and turn quickly back to look at the person. Never change your facial expression. In many cases you will see that the direct eye contact you made the first time has made the other person feel uncomfortable and that when you look the second time he will look away or put his head down.

Your eyes create a first impression, and the more confidence and defensiveness you project, the less likely you are to become the target of a Bad Guy who would prefer to prey on the weak.

Eyes on the Sides of Your Head

Several years ago I provided protection for Senator Bill Bradley when he went to a book signing following the publication of his autobiography. After the signing, I and another member of the protection team accompanied the senator to a luncheon where he was to be the speaker. During his speech, he spoke briefly about having trained his eyes to look forward but to see also what was going on to either side. He said that having trained his peripheral vision had helped him to play better basketball.

Thinking about it, I realized that many attacks or abduction attempts come from our "blind spots," either from behind or from the side, and I went back to the mall to work on my own technique. To improve your side vision, walk through a mall when it is least crowded, which is generally during the week, in the morning or midafternoon, when most people are at work. As you walk, concentrate on looking straight ahead, but try to see what is on either side of you. Start by identifying colors, then objects, then the signs over individual shops. As you develop your peripheral vision, you will become able to open your car door and see who is to the side of you without indicating that you are aware he is there.

At speaking engagements, I look at someone in the audience and tell him what someone on the opposite end of the room is doing, just to demonstrate that self-preservation is more a training of the senses than it is learning hand-to-hand combat.

Reading a Walk

- *The Carefree Walk*. This is the gait of someone whose mind is elsewhere, who's taking his time, and who might unintentionally bump into other people or objects because he's not thinking about what he's doing, and then apologize immediately. In most cases this is perfectly harmless behavior, so just be on your guard and, should you spot someone like this walking toward you, say, "Excuse me," loudly enough to get the person's focus back to reality. In most cases he or she will say "I'm sorry," and move aside.

- *The Distressed Walk*. This is the fast, frantic walk of someone weaving in and out among other pedestrians because he's in a rush to arrive at his destination. You see this walk every day on city streets because people are so focused on their destination that they are oblivious of their surroundings. It's a walk that indicates either stress or frustration—or both. People who walk this walk are often concentrating on an upsetting or emergency situation. When I spot this type of walk, I just step aside and allow the person to pass.

- *The Confrontational Walk*. This is the stride of the person who wants to let you know he is in charge. He'll walk directly toward you, expecting you to get out of his way. He might even walk in front of your car when you have the right of way, just challenging you to run him down. He's not happy with who he is, and is therefore trying to prove himself every day and in every way—especially at someone else's expense. He may also be looking for a scapegoat—someone he can use to inflate his own ego or on whom he can release his tensions. When you spot someone like this, stay away. Should he confront you, make your way into a store or some other public area and let it be known that this person is harassing you. Bring attention to the situation as soon as possible.

- *The Lost Walk.* Stopping, looking, hesitating, then moving on, this is the walk of a frustrated person trying to find his way. He's probably in an area that's unfamiliar to him or has temporarily lost his bearings. This person usually means no harm. If someone like this should approach you and you don't want to help, just say, "I'm sorry, I'm not familiar with this area," and keep on walking. If you want to be helpful, don't give directions, but steer the person to someone in a position of authority, such as a security guard. Personally, I never stop when I'm with my family because their safety always comes first.

- *The Protective Walk.* This is the scanning, observing walk of the person who plans ahead and takes the safest route. He's usually half a pace slower than anyone he's with, and generally walks close to the wall, to the side of a staircase, or wherever he is likely to encounter the least pedestrian traffic. These people don't become a problem to anyone unless you create the problem yourself. It is also the walk you want to assume yourself. As I've said before, first impressions are all-important, and if you look like you fit into the area and are aware of your surroundings, you'll be a less attractive target.

Reading What We "Say" When We're Seated

- *Relaxed Position.* Legs comfortable, mind distracted, talking on the phone or reading the newspaper. You see people sitting this way in airports or other waiting areas and riding mass transit. It's the position of people who are often caught off guard and have their purses or laptops stolen. It's all well and good to be comfortable, but staying alert will keep you secure.

- *Tense Position.* Hands in constant motion, chest puffed out, eyes staring. It's a position that lets you know the person is on edge and looking for confrontation just to release his hostilities. You see people sitting this way when they're too hot or too cold, or when they're jammed into crowded quarters. If you see someone broadcasting his tension your way, you don't want to risk antagonizing him. Limit your eye contact and avoid getting into a conversation.

- *Fidgety Position.* Eyes and body in constant motion. Can't get comfortable. Keeps getting up and sitting down. People fidget for many different, usually innocent reasons. The fidgety person may be uncomfortable in his seat (such as those molded plastic chairs you find in airports), his clothing may be too tight, or he may have eaten too much. This person is generally not looking for a confrontation. More likely, he will eventually find his comfort zone and remain in that position until it's time to move on.

- *"Zoned Out" Position.* Staring at the ceiling or the floor. Mind focused inward. Doesn't have a clue or a care about what's going on. Usually the person in this position is lost in thought and has completely forgotten about the world around him. He may be focusing on some deep-seated problem of his own. His obliviousness, however, can lead to unpredictable random or impulsive movements. And, depending upon what's on his mind, he may or may not be volatile. Avoid conversation and prolonged eye contact at all costs.

- *Secure Position.* Comfortable yet alert. Eyes scanning. Stretches legs periodically to prevent them from becoming stiff or cramped. This position indicates that the person is on "standby alert" both mentally and physically. It's the position that allows so many "civilians" to spot a police officer or a member of the military simply by his appearance. People who sit this way are usually trained in the protective services or some kind of high-level security. In most cases they're good people to have around, and it's all right to observe them because they have already observed you.

Learning the language of position and expression means not only that you'll be more likely to recognize a potentially violent, dangerous, or simply confrontational person when you see one, but also that you'll be able to adjust your own body language so that you'll be less likely to be targeted as a victim.

Several years ago, I was hired by Fox TV to protect one of their then-upcoming stars, a teenager named David Faustino, who played

LEARN HOW AND WHEN TO END A CONVERSATION

As I've already said, some of us "good guys" are just too polite when it comes to ending a conversation with a stranger, even when our best instincts are telling us the person we're stuck talking to is really a creep.

If you want to do it the polite way, here are a couple of suggestions. Glance at your watch and say, "Oh my goodness, I'm late. Nice meeting you. 'Bye!" Or you can say, "Excuse me, but I have to go call my husband [or wife]; he [or she] is waiting for me and I'm already late."

If, on the other hand, you don't care so much about being polite to a stranger, just say "Excuse me," and leave.

TOM'S TIP

the role of Bud Bundy on the hit show *Married With Children*. Dave met with me, Todd Parisi, who was one of my most trusted colleagues, and members of his own organization to discuss his security needs. We built a very strong professional relationship and provided him with security coverage for the next several years.

On one occasion, Dave asked us to take him to a teen club, and, since there were none at the time in New Jersey, we did some advance work and found one in Rockland County, New York. Dave approved the choice, and we took him to the club, where he was recognized and greeted by virtually everyone who saw him, and lines of young girls waited to get his autograph. The club was open to anyone eighteen years of age or older, and those who were over twenty-one could purchase alcoholic beverages. One particular girl kept coming over and flirting with Dave, who responded politely and professionally. At one point the girl mentioned that her boyfriend was getting mad, and after she left to go back to him, I made eye contact and could see the fire in his eyes as he spoke to her.

As the evening progressed, I kept him in my direct line of sight and observed that he was drinking excessively. The last time she came over to our table, she got Dave's autograph and then kissed him on the cheek, wrote her phone number on a napkin, and gave it to him. Just as she did that, her enraged boyfriend grabbed a beer bottle and stormed across the dance floor. I told Todd to get Dave out of the club, and made a beeline for the boyfriend. We met midway across the dance floor, and he was so focused on Dave that he never saw me coming. I applied a CDT restraint, relieved him of the beer bottle, and ushered him over to the exit, where the bouncers helped me remove him from the premises.

Once he was outside, I left him to the bouncers and made my way to our car, where Todd, the driver, and Dave were waiting. As I slid into my seat, I asked Dave if he was okay. "I didn't even know there was a problem," he replied. "How did you know?"

"His eyes gave him away," I said, "and his aggressive walk confirmed it."

TRAINING FOR LIFE: INCREASING YOUR ODDS THROUGH MENTAL AND PHYSICAL CONDITIONING

As I've been emphasizing throughout this book, preparation is the key to success in virtually any situation. And preparation does not mean simply keeping yourself physically fit or mentally alert; it requires a combination of the two. Physically, it means learning a few simple and specific techniques that use common, everyday motions like turning a key, knocking on a door, and clapping your hands. These are the techniques we teach in CDT training and which I'll be describing in the next chapter. It also means training your mind to process your perceptions quickly and accurately. To maximize the odds that you'll emerge unharmed from a potentially violent situation, your body and mind must work together as a cohesive unit.

Physical Training

If we were to believe what we see on television and read in popular magazines, we'd have to think that learning karate or jujitsu or some other form of martial arts will turn us into physically fit, well-oiled fighting machines. The truth, however, is that not all of us are capable of becoming Chuck Norris, and learning martial arts in a training center is very different from being able to apply those skills in a real-life situation. In addition, the martial arts are more about combat and fighting than about personal protection.

I would prefer that my clients learn the kinds of skills that will make it less likely they'll ever have to fight, because the average person doesn't fight, though he can get into altercations or violent situations. If you can avoid a fight, you'll be sure to avoid getting hurt. Hence the name Training for Life. The real key to Training for Life lies not in toning your muscles but in conditioning your mind. It's about brains, not brawn, about how to outsmart the bad guy as simply and safely as possible, not how to beat him up.

A young woman in one of my awareness classes told me a story about how brainpower had worked for her. She'd been dating a bodybuilder who was preparing for a competition. As part of his training regimen he used unauthorized steroids to enhance his physique and build his strength and power. That was something he thought he had to do because he wasn't as big as most of the other competitors. The drugs, however, caused him to have violent mood swings known as " 'roid rages" and on one particular occasion, the woman told me, he just "flipped out" while they were in the parking lot of a shopping center. The argument started because they were deciding where to eat, and her boyfriend became so angry that he grabbed her by the throat and demanded that she drive him to a sushi restaurant.

As soon as he let her go, she agreed. She asked him to please put her shopping bag in the trunk, indicating that she would get in the car and unlock it from the inside. She started the car, and as her boyfriend was walking around to the back, she stepped on the gas and left him literally holding the bag.

Then, still feeling insulted, aggravated, and violated, she drove directly to the police station and filed assault charges. Her boyfriend was picked up while he was still in the parking lot trying to figure out how to get home. In the end she dropped the charges, but did take out a restraining order against him.

She learned one of the most important lessons we teach in Training for Life, which is to use whatever method of distraction is at your disposal even if it means allowing the Bad Guy to believe you're intimidated and, most of all, not to worry about material possessions but always to put safety first.

Mental Training

Whenever we find ourselves in a difficult situation, one with which we're unfamiliar, or one for which we're unprepared, we will naturally experience some level of self-doubt. When that situation is volatile, any kind of doubt will delay our physical reactions and can therefore turn potential victory into tragic defeat.

The best way to minimize doubt is to maximize preparation. In my career as an international protection specialist, I've spent many hours traveling to jobs, and I use most of that travel time mentally rehearsing every situation I can imagine occurring and developing a variety of scenarios for potential courses of action. My philosophy is that everyone should always prepare for the worst and hope for the best. That doesn't mean I think you ought to be spending your life dreaming up worst-case scenarios or preparing for violence; I am suggesting, however, that training your senses and developing mental resiliency will serve you well when your biology throws you into fight-or-flight and your brain involuntarily begins to play tricks on you.

Years ago, when my schedule was less hectic and time wasn't so scarce, I used to work out on Sundays at the various martial arts schools with which I was associated. After training we all would go to breakfast or lunch, depending on the time. One day a group of guys from South Jersey came to the workout. One man with whom I was working out, a guy named Jerry, told me that he didn't know how well he would fare in a street fight. He said he'd always been afraid that if he ever hit someone in self-defense he'd hold back because he didn't really want to hurt him. If he did that, he said, he wasn't sure whether his attacker would learn a lesson or whether he'd just get mad. Then he went on to tell me that when he was driving, or if he just had some idle time, he often wondered what a street fight would be like, and sometimes he saw himself as the victim rather than the defender.

He asked about my profession and what violence is really like in a real-life altercation. I told him that violence is an animal that takes on different shapes. Just like people, I said, no two altercations are alike. I did tell him, however, that if negative thoughts were with him now, they'd be with him when and if he met an attacker head-on. What he needed to do, I added, was to conquer those negative thoughts by having confidence in his training and his ability to defend himself.

Then I told him about another guy I knew, named John, who was a martial arts black belt and who'd gotten into a fight at a rest stop located off the Garden State Parkway, in New Jersey. What happened was that a burly guy the size of an NFL linebacker had made some comment to John's girlfriend about her rear end. When the guy began to get graphic about what he wanted to do to her, John stepped in. The big guy pushed John first; then John stepped back, threw a front kick to his groin, and missed. The guy looked at him, charged him head-on, picked him up by his waist, body-slammed him to the ground, and proceeded to hit him repeatedly. That's when two men who happened to be off-duty Delaware police officers intervened and subdued the man until the state police arrived. John was rushed to the hospital with broken ribs, a fractured skull, and numerous broken bones in his face.

When I went to see him in the hospital, he was a truly shaken man. "Tom," he said, "you're right. Once a negative thought gets into your head, you're finished. And once I missed that first kick, the negative thoughts just took over."

In fairness to John, it wasn't only the negative thoughts that sabotaged him but also the type of training he did. He practiced a martial art that taught controlled fighting, which means that you pull your blows and don't make any type of contact when you spar. The problem was that his muscle memory kicked in and he pulled his kick so that instead of really hitting the target area, which was the groin, he just tapped it, which, of course, gave the big guy the opportunity to wreak havoc with John's mind and body.

John has since dropped out of the martial arts, and the last time we spoke, which was many years ago, he still seemed not to have recovered from the emotional scarring left by that tragic event.

VIOLENCE IN THE STREETS: HOW IT REALLY HAPPENS

If you've already had the misfortune to be confronted by someone who wanted to harm you, you'll know the truth of the mental and physical reactions I'm about to describe. If you've been lucky enough to avoid this kind of confrontation, my description will help you to understand why it's so important to be prepared in advance for the chaos your biology will wreak on your mind and body.

The body and mind of the person accustomed to living with violence will react differently from the body and mind of the one who is not. Let's first talk about the unseasoned, untrained person—the majority of the population. When violence shatters the peaceful mindset of the average person, his body begins to react in certain ways. Peripheral vision shuts down and he can see only straight ahead. Tunnel vision becomes a reality rather than a figure of speech. His breathing becomes rapid, his heart pounds, and that internal "noise" prevents him from hearing external sounds. His stomach knots and his legs begin to feel like jelly. His hands are tense and their movement agitated. In some cases he may lose control of his bodily functions; his eyes may tear and his bowels release. His body falls prey to the fear that has taken over his mind.

A trained person, on the other hand, one who has experienced real violence on more than one occasion, reacts quite differently. The eyes refocus so that he is looking through, rather than directly at, his attacker. He is taking in not only what is directly in front of him but the surrounding area as well. His hearing becomes sharper, picking up every sound and distinguishing between those that signal danger and those that do not. His breathing is more rapid but still under control. His heart beats more rapidly to increase blood flow, not out of nervousness but to prepare his body for its defense. His stance shifts so that he is standing in profile to the attacker, protecting his vital organs, while his arms lock into a defensive position and his hands remain relaxed.

The seasoned defender doesn't think about what he has to do; his body and mind are disciplined to respond automatically to subconscious instinct and muscle memory. Fear is not a factor.

One also needs to understand that for some people—especially for those who use it for the wrong reasons—violence is a stimulant, a rush, the highest of highs. Most of the world doesn't know what it's like to be able to hurt or even kill another person. The key to success for many Bad Guys is their attitude, which is, simply put, "You may want to hurt me, but I will kill you." And, in all fairness, they're right, because there are very few average citizens who can beat them at their own game.

That's why I continue to tell people that it doesn't happen the way they think, and that if for any reason they find themselves in a violent encounter with a Bad Guest or a Bad Guy, the key to survival is to escape as quickly as possible. To do that, you need to pay attention to what's going on around you, deal with the moment, and not worry about why you, of all people, are being victimized.

The majority of bad situations take time to develop, which means there are always windows of opportunity for escape, but those windows shut and remain shut when you lack training. Most people's threshold of pain is extremely low—a few harsh words and a good slap in the face will begin the process of intimidation. Understand that the body wants to live and will preserve itself in any way it can, but it needs help. It needs to be educated, updated, and trained to be aware and take advantage of every viable option for getting away from a violent situation as quickly as possible.

In the following chapter, I'll offer specific recommendations for various types of training and help you to begin your own training at home with my own revolutionary personal protection skills called Training for Life using the CDT system. This system, as I've already said, is both easy to learn and easy to remember. I developed it originally for the people I care about but can't be with every minute of the day, and now I'm passing it along to you. So put aside whatever negative thoughts you may have had about your ability to protect yourself. Your life is about to change for the better.

SIX

BE PREPARED—THE CDT WAY

PHASE ONE. *It's cold and dark and you're walking alone in an unfamiliar area. You come to a dark side street, and just as you turn the corner, the unthinkable happens. Your worst nightmare. A man steps out of the shadows and utters a cold, direct threat. Before you can utter a sound, his hands are at your throat, squeezing the life out of you.*

YOUR REACTION. *Your emotions are a mix of self-pity, fear, and anger. You're struggling with the "why me?" syndrome. You want to run and hide, but you can't. Suddenly you realize that this is the test of your life, and you begin to take control of your emotions and gather your senses. This is a do-or-die moment, and you know it. You feel weak and drained of energy, but you begin to gather your inner strength as your will to live kicks in. You've just passed the first test!*

PHASE TWO. *Your attacker takes one hand from your throat and hits you in the face, knocking you momentarily senseless. You might begin to cry, and then you become enraged because this person has violated your personal innocence. Because you've taken the steps to acquire and practice Training for Life skills, your mind is now working and your body is getting ready to fight back. Your mind is* *saying, "I am the protector of my own life and I will do what I have to in order to survive." You strike hard and fast. Your attacker loosens his grip and stumbles to the ground. For a moment you don't quite know what to do. You want to laugh and cry at the same time. Then you turn and run for help. You've passed the test of survival, and the prize is your life!*

YOU MAY NOT yet have encountered violence in the streets, but if you've learned the skills of Training for Life and the worst should occur, your training will give you the ability to protect yourself. The above scenario provides a pretty clear picture of how such an event might unfold. But why Training for Life and learning CDT techniques rather than following one of the more traditional so-called self-protection programs that have been on the scene much longer? Let's take a look at the options, which generally involve some form of the martial arts.

THE MARTIAL ARTS: WHAT EXACTLY ARE THEY, AND HOW DO THEY WORK?

We've all probably seen at least one action movie or TV program in which a ninja-like martial artist takes on a group of deadly attackers and vanquishes them all with a series of well-placed kicks, chops, and blows. How does he do that? Is it realistic? Could the average person really perform that way?

I've been involved in various forms of martial-arts training since I was a small boy. I still do them today and have incorporated their practice into my personal belief system, so I can give you a pretty good idea of how they vary from one form to another, and what to expect from each one. Many years ago, the only systems taught were the traditional forms, including aikido, karate, kung fu, which is among the most ancient, judo, jujitsu, and, the most widely taught of all, tae kwon do.

For most of their history, the roots and techniques of each of these systems were passed down from one master to another without ever changing or updating it in any way. More recently, however, various instructors have broken away from these traditions, combining two or more systems to create an entirely new one, putting their personal stamp on the program they've "invented." Today there are well over 3,000 hybrid versions of the martial arts being taught. In some ways, such innovation has diluted the integrity of the original forms, but it has also rejuvenated the arts by mixing and matching techniques that would never have been taught together before.

Traditional Martial Arts

The traditional combative arts originated in China and Japan during feudal times, and are generally based upon specific fighting techniques that follow preset patterns of movement known as *kata* or forms. They emphasize not only conditioning the body but also training the "warrior" mind to defend against all types of armed and unarmed attack.

One of the most positive aspects of traditional martial-arts training is that it teaches us to view the body as a temple to be protected and preserved at all cost. In its purest form, it teaches humility and honor backed by courage, respect, and, most of all, discipline. On the negative side, many of the traditional techniques are too outdated, too rigid, and in some cases too barbaric either to be appealing or to be practical in real-life situations.

Fewer than ten percent of those teaching martial arts today follow these traditional forms because, on the one hand, most people simply don't have the degree of self-discipline needed to learn them correctly, and, on the other, many martial-arts classes are directed to children, for whom the environment in one of these sessions would be much too strict. Anyone interested in learning a traditional form of the martial arts would do well to start either with hard-style karate, which originated in Japan; tae kwon do, which originated in Korea; or hard- or soft-style kung fu, which originated in China.

Sporting-Oriented Martial Arts

The most popular of the traditional sporting arts are karate, tae kwon do, and judo. Karate is based on wide, strong stances along with direct punching and kicking. Tae kwon do is an art that teaches a dominance of feet over hands. It depends on multiple power kicks developed from every possible angle, both in a straight line and spinning. Watching a tae kwon do expert is like watching poetry in motion. Judo is a system that depends on speed and power combined with leverage. It depends on your being light on your feet and able to offset the weight of your opponent.

Judo, in fact, was the first form of martial-arts sport fighting to be accepted as an official Olympic event. Its popularity increased in the United States when Mike Swain won the gold medal at the World Games and then went on to compete in the Olympics. Mike is a pioneer in the martial arts who is totally dedicated to his sport. Unfortunately, however, judo has been losing popularity in the last several years, mainly because it isn't as flashy as some other forms and because it involves choking and constantly being thrown to the mat, which take a heavy toll on the body. Judo is a sport that can easily be adapted for self-defense, but it requires a lot of time to learn well.

Combative Martial Arts

In recent years, many of the old, traditional martial arts have given way to "new" or "eclectic" forms that mix a variety of styles or techniques. In fact, boxing and wrestling techniques are now being used in many modern martial-arts schools for what is known as cross-training, which means, in effect, combining a variety of fighting styles to come up with the ultimate arsenal.

Arts based on military or government training have been particularly intriguing to teenagers and young adults aged about fourteen to twenty-four, who enroll in these courses to become overnight Green Berets only to discover, several weeks later, that they hate it and move on to some other faddish form of training.

In some cases these new forms can, however, be extremely positive and useful. As with so many things we learn, it depends on the integrity and intent of the person who is teaching it. Richard Faustini is one martial artist whose talent and intent are both admirable. A few years ago, Rich broke his ties to the traditional arts to start Heiho Shin Do, an eclectic system based on some tradition, some sport, and very sound combative defense. When he first went out on his own, he was ridiculed just as I was when I started CDT. Now, however, his school in Oradell, New Jersey, is flourishing. Like most martial-arts schools, his includes a high percentage of children in its enrollment, and the parents I've spoken to all praise him for stressing the importance of education, respect for the parents, honesty in one's daily activities, and just being a good human being. They speak of him as a positive role model, which is what all modern teachers of martial arts should be aiming for.

Not everyone will be comfortable with these more eclectic systems, but that doesn't make them right or wrong, it just makes them more set in their ways.

Why Don't More People Learn Martial Arts?

In the course of my Training for Life seminars, I've spoken to many people from all walks of life about why they haven't learned—or have stopped training in—some form of the martial arts. Since one of my goals is to educate them about personal defense in general and how the arts could be a positive force in their overall training, I wanted to know why they stayed away. These are the reasons they most commonly gave:

Too Time-Consuming Like any other athletic skill, such as skiing, golfing, or tennis, learning a martial art requires that you commit time to both mastering and practicing its techniques. There are, however, schools that offer forty-five-minute classes rather than the more traditional ninety-minute sessions in order to accommodate people with only a limited amount of free time. Another alternative might be to make this an activity in which the entire family participates by taking a class on weekends. Practicing even once a week is better than never practicing at all!

Preexisting Injuries People often tell me they have a bad back or a bad knee or a chronic health problem such as asthma and therefore can't do this kind of training. My response is that before you begin any kind of physical-training program, you should consult with your own physician. But most good martial-arts schools will work with your limitations and might even help to strengthen a bad back or a bad knee. Unqualified schools or poor instruction might, of course, cause further damage. So check out the school carefully before you join, but realize as well that having a preexisting condition is not an excuse for failing to learn to defend yourself. If you run into a Bad Guy on the street, he isn't going to know—or care—that you have a bad back!

My oldest brother, Phil, is ten years my senior and one of my closest friends. When I began teaching martial arts at the Lodi Boys Club, he became one of my first students. He'd damaged his knee very badly in a skiing accident, but despite his injury he trained as hard as anyone else, if not harder. I was pretty tough in those days, and sometimes the workouts would exacerbate his condition. But I was also relentless, telling him, "The guy on the street isn't going to care if you're hurt. He'll finish you right there if you give up."

Then one evening Phil and I and a group of our friends were invited to a bachelor party at a club in New York City. We took a limo into town so that we'd be able to drink and not worry about driving home. As it turned out, one of my friends was dancing with a young woman whose ex-boyfriend apparently decided he wanted her back. An argument broke out on the dance floor, and the bouncer decided to remove both our group and the other guy's. When I got outside, I could see that the argument was intensifying, and I decided to become the mediator. I apologized to the other group for the misunderstanding and suggested that we all go to another bar where the drinks would be on us. My plan was that while they headed for the bar, we'd get in the limo and go to a club in New Jersey where we were known.

It seemed as if things were going well when one of their guys got a little bit too antsy and punched one of our guys in the face, knocking him to the ground. That's when all hell broke loose. We were outnumbered, and it was every man for himself. My immediate reaction was to hit hard, hit fast, and then look out for my brother. When I found him, it looked as if he were wedged between two cars, and as I got closer, I could see that he was holding on to the bumper of a van and defending himself with one hand and one foot. One guy was already unconscious on the ground to his right, and just as I got close enough to help, he knocked out a second one as well.

I could see from his eyes that Phil was in pain, and when I looked at his knee, I could see it was obviously dislocated. Apparently he'd slipped on the wet pavement, but instead of giving up, he'd set his mind to defend himself. He proved to me that night that anyone, no matter what his limitations, can defend himself so long as he has good training and the will to survive.

It Doesn't Work Well, that's sometimes true, but it isn't necessarily the fault of the training or of the art being taught. The latter is only one part of the equation; the mindset of the student is the other. We are a society made up of mainly good people while the criminals who intend to hurt us are bad people, and, in an altercation, that can be a problem. In most cases, however, it isn't the art that fails, it's the person. I've worked with people who had no training at all but who fought with the strength of a bear and the fury of a tiger, and they fared very well in a fight. But I've also worked with some black belts who didn't fare well at all.

I first met Tom Carrillo, the head of security for Fox TV in New York City, in 1989, when he invited me to come to his office to discuss whether my newly formed company could do some work for the network. At the time, New York was in turmoil following the Bensonhurst riots, which broke out after a white male teenager shot and killed a black male teenager. When we met, Tom explained that Fox was having problems with camera people and reporters being assaulted while on assignment, and his boss, vice-president Tony Fragetti, wanted to provide a better-trained security force for their personnel.

Other security firms had apparently refused to take the assignment. In fact, he told me that their previous team of bodyguards had been so scared when violence broke out that they'd run to the safety of the van and left the client, a news reporter, out on the street alone. I, however, was eager for the work and had faith in the men I employed, so I agreed to do the job. I split my men up into teams of two and took for my partner the newest member of our organization, a martial artist who owned his own school and, at least in a classroom environment, seemed to know what he was doing.

Our first assignment was working with Penny Crone, a dedicated reporter who would do anything to get to the heart of a story. When we met, she said she'd received a tip and that we were going to Harlem to interview a relative of the deceased black teenager. When we arrived at the location, the air was filled with tension and the crowd was hostile—very hostile. Another news channel had apparently done a story the community considered less than accurate, and they were not happy to see us.

After about five minutes we'd made no progress and the name-calling appeared to be escalating, so I decided to get Ms. Crone back in the van and get out of there. As we started to leave, however, three very large African-American men stood in front of the vehicle, making it impossible for us to move. At that point I said to my partner, "Let's clear the way," and we both got out of the van. As I approached the men blocking the way, I said, "Guys, we're not here to cause problems. We're just doing our jobs and we'd like to leave the neighborhood in peace. If we've offended anyone in any way, we certainly apologize." That was my first and last attempt at diplomacy. The leader of the group put his face directly in mine and stared. He was so close that I could actually hear his heart pounding. This went on for what probably was a minute, but it felt more like an hour. I was conditioned for this, however, and my mindset switched immediately from that of a diplomat to that of a defender. Then, just as quickly as the guy had gotten in my face, he moved away and walked over to my partner.

He stared at the new guy who was acting as my partner, then glanced back at me and said, "I'm cool with you. We have no problems." My partner, however, was starting to sweat, and then he made his big mistake; he looked away from the guy who was staring at him and said, "I don't want any problems." That opened the floodgates. The three guys began to ridicule and spit at my red-headed partner until I pulled him by his jacket and shoved him back into the van. I then stood in front of the vehicle as I asked point-blank, "Are you going to move or do we have to go to the next level?" The leader just smirked and said, "Man, get yourself a new partner." I extended my hand and he extended his. We shook. Then he turned to his guys and said, "It's cool."

After the detail was over and we were on our way home, I asked my partner if he was all right. He looked at me and said, "Tom, I never realized what this profession was about. In my school, I'm the master, but I learned today that means nothing on the street. I give you credit for what you do, but it's not for me."

Being trained is a good thing, but unless your mindset matches your training, intimidation will wreak havoc with your mind and body. The street can be a hard place to learn a lesson, and the lesson can be very humbling.

It's Too Expensive It's only too expensive if you're not getting what you think you've paid for. Teaching martial arts is big business, and, as in any other business, there are quality vendors and those who are not. To be a smart consumer, you first need to educate yourself about the school itself. Ask the following questions:

1. How long has it been in business?

2. Is it properly insured, and by whom?

3. Do all instructors go through criminal history checks, and, if so, can

you see the report? If the answer to the first question is no, find another school. If the answer to the second is no, ask why not.

4. What is the reputation of the school in the community?

5. What are the fees, and are there any hidden charges you should know about before you sign up?

6. What kinds of programs are being taught?

7. If I sign up (or enroll my child) and it turns out that the program is not right for me (or the child), is there a period of time during which I can cancel the contract without being charged the full fee?

If you've asked all the questions, and the school delivers on its promises, don't blame the program if, two weeks later, you decide to drop out. These schools are businesses and they deserve to be paid for their services, so do the right thing and make those payments.

I Hate the Whole Environment A place of learning should, I believe, be representative of the material being taught, and it's no different whether the material is martial arts or medicine. Calling an instructor "sir," "ma'am," or *sensei* in the Japanese arts, *sifu* in the Chinese arts, *guro* in the Filipino arts, or *sabumnim* in the Korean arts is no different from calling a doctor or professor by his or her title. It may take some getting used to, but these instructors have earned their rank, and using their titles is part of the discipline of the art. I do believe, however, that the use of these courtesy titles ought to remain within the walls of the training facility. Taking advantage of one's title can lead to behavior that reflects badly on the martial arts as a whole. I saw that behavior firsthand when, shortly after I opened my school, the owner of another local school, a guy named John, invited me to dinner. We went to a local Italian restaurant and he seemed like a nice enough, fairly easygoing guy, except that he told me he wanted to be addressed as "Master." When I let him know that wasn't going to happen, we agreed to disagree. While we were eating, however, two of John's students came into the restaurant and stopped by our table several times, always addressing him as "Master" and asking if there was anything he needed. Then, when I asked for the check, our waiter informed me that the Master's students had picked up our tab. I told him that I appreciated the gesture but I preferred to pay my own way. Master John, however, stated that his students had been told that anytime they saw him in a restaurant, either alone or with a guest, it was their duty to pay his bill. I just looked at him and said, "You have got to be kidding!"

"You run your school your way, and I'll run mine" was his reply.

Needless to say, I never had dinner with Master John again.

It's Too Hard to Learn As is true for other kinds of physical training, it may take a while for you to figure out what your body is capable of and what it is not. Whether it's a soft style like tai chi, a kicking system like tae kwon do, a hard style like karate, or a combative style like Hom-Do, it has to be compatible with your particular body and mindset if it is to work for you. But just because you enter one kind of program and it doesn't seem to fit doesn't mean you should give up on the martial arts completely. In my opinion, lately too much emphasis has been placed on the combative forms, and because the average person is not conditioned for combat, he or she will enroll and then become disenchanted after the first few classes.

A friend of mine had learned an overseas combat system and added it to the curriculum of his school. In the first week of advertising the new program, forty new students signed up; two weeks later, thirty-two of them had dropped out. What my friend had forgotten was that he was teaching average Joes and Janes, not Navy SEALs. He's now simplified the system and offers it as a form of cardiovascular training for women. He added some music, some drills of his own devising, cut the length of the workout from an hour to thirty minutes, and allows his students to break for a glass of water whenever they want. It's been a great success because he's brought the demands of the program into line with the abilities and desires of his students. In addition, he is very honest with people who join his classes, telling them that his system is a combative martial art that teaches physical fitness, not self-defense in the street.

The Martial Arts Are Just for Kids

I've already discussed some of the positive and negative aspects of martial-arts training for children, but the fact remains that if you consider "adult" to begin at the age of eighteen, there are, in fact, approximately eight children for every adult enrolled in martial-arts classes. In many schools, children and adults attend classes together.

Because the curriculum is based upon expertise, not age, children are expected to learn the same material as adults on their level. Nevertheless, working with adults is not necessarily the best thing for the children, as I discovered when I was eight years old and taking aikido, the first of the martial arts that I studied. I was a blue belt at the time, and sparring with an older man who kicked me right in the eye. It was close to the end of the class, so my father had just walked in to pick me up, and there I was on the floor, my face and eye full of blood. I was a tough kid, and I would have gotten up to finish the sparring, despite the fact that my eye was full of a combination of blood and tears. The instructor, however, intervened, stopped the sparring, and got someone to attend to my eye. At that point my father stepped in, looked at my eye, and announced that he was taking me to the hospital and would be back to talk with the head instructor the next day. I don't know what he said, but from that day on, adults and children were taught separately. Meanwhile, it took six stitches to sew up my eye. I still have the scar.

I suggest that if you prefer to work in a class that includes only adults, you make that clear to your instructor. And if you do work in a mixed class, I suggest that children work with children and adults with adults. The fact is that because the student body at most martial-arts schools is skewed toward children, there will, more often than not, be children taking classes with adults.

Government Regulation—Good or Bad?

Recently the federal government has been looking into the possibility of regulating the teaching of martial arts. But, as I've already said, there are now so many styles and so many systems, based on so many different philosophies and cultures, that this would be very difficult to do. Mel Klein, a good friend of mine who owns a martial-arts supply shop in Emerson, New Jersey, spends a great deal of his own time and money advocating against regulation, not because it would adversely affect his business but because he is a dedicated martial artist and wants the arts to remain free. Like many others, he believes that the martial arts teach creativity, integrity, respect, and humility, as well as perpetuating the ideas and philosophies of the styles' founders. To him, the martial arts are a form of self-expression, and he firmly believes that one ought to have the freedom to choose how one wishes to express oneself.

I believe that because there are so many styles, schools, and systems, even with some form of regulation it would be difficult if not impossible to control those who operate what I call fly-by-night operations out of their own homes or through the martial-arts "underground." And, unfortunately, those are exactly the people who are responsible for making regulation a possibility.

Last year I went to a meeting of people on both sides of the question. Those in favor of regulation wanted to run background checks on all instructors and to close all schools that didn't carry liability and medical insurance. Those who were against regulation claimed it would infringe upon their First Amendment rights to freedom of expression. Both sides had stories to tell in support of their position.

Personally, I have studied both the traditional and "renegade" forms of martial arts, and it's my belief that martial artists can no more be expected to conform to general standards that limit their freedom of expression than can musicians, painters, sculptors, or dancers. I do think, however, that before one is awarded a license to teach, one should have to undergo a background check, as do private detectives, other kinds of teachers, and security personnel. What one chooses to teach should be one's own business, so long as it falls within the guidelines of a traditional, sporting, combative, or personal defense art. I also believe that anyone who operates a school should be required to check the background of anyone he or she hires to teach, and that schools should be required to carry insurance for medical or liability claims. While the "artistic" aspect of the arts requires freedom to thrive, the business side ought to be subject to some specific regulation.

Like anything else you set out to buy, learn, or participate in, you are primarily responsible for doing the job of investigating the product and making sure not only that you're getting your money's worth but also that you're "buying" something that will be useful and that you'll be happy to live with over time.

If you have the mindset, the dedication, and the physical skills, this kind of training can be extremely useful in helping you learn to protect yourself. Unfortunately—and realistically—however, I've found that very few people are willing to devote either the time or the energy that is required to master these arts. And, in addition, it's very difficult for the average citizen to put into practice what he's learned in a controlled, safe environment when he's suddenly confronted by a bad guy on the street.

SELF-DEFENSE COURSES

As I've traveled around the country speaking to various groups, one thing I've discovered is that many people, at some time in their lives—usually their late teens or early twenties—have taken some kind of self-protection course. Such courses are given in community centers, gyms, high schools, and sometimes even elementary schools. The classes are generally an hour long, held once a week, and last for eight weeks.

Critics of these self-defense classes make a good argument that many of the strategies they emphasize are designed for stranger-assault situations rather than for the more common scenarios such as date rape, encountering a Bad Guest, or a basic pushing and shoving match that's intended to demonstrate toughness but not to do deadly harm. And, in fact, the philosophy behind most self-defense *is* to "defend at all cost" and "annihilate the attacker." Most people with whom I've spoken who had taken one of these courses told me they'd dropped out after the first few weeks because they got bored, because they were unable to master the moves that were being taught, or because the idea of hurting or maiming another person—even in self-defense—was not only against their nature but also against their better judgment. Many of them added that they thought the classes were being treated as some kind of alternative singles bar, with the instructor more interested in showing off than in teaching the techniques, and the students more interested in talking about where they'd be going for dinner than in learning them.

When I asked what kinds of techniques were included in the course, virtually everyone said they'd been taught to take out the eyes, to throw a punch or chop to the throat, and to kick or grab the groin. When I asked how many of them remembered anything they'd been taught, the room invariably fell silent. And when I asked if any of them thought they'd be able to tear out someone else's eyes, they all shook their heads, and their body language said "No way."

Back in the early 1980s, I was hired to teach my first corporate self-defense class. When I arrived the first day, there were forty students in the room. Since the company employed several hundred, I thought that was a pretty small turnout. But, looking back, in light of the fact that there was very little interest among the general population in either the martial arts or self-defense at that time, I guess it wasn't bad.

In any case, my attitude at the time was that most of the people in this world were soft and needed to toughen up, so I ran my class like a drill sergeant. My mission was to "get through to them," because, to my mind, I was from the real world and they worked behind the corporate wall. The first thing I did was a drill to see how many push-ups and sit-ups each of my "students" could do. I wasn't ready for what I discovered. Most of them couldn't do ten push-ups even when they were cheating, and even fewer could do fifteen sit-ups. My next test was to ask everyone to stand on one leg for thirty seconds; most of them dropped their other leg in fewer than twelve. The next and final test was to have them go face-to-face with a partner and stare into each other's eyes for one minute as if they were facing a seasoned adversary. That test lasted for fewer than twenty seconds. At that point my fellow instructor, who held a black belt in karate, and I looked at each other and said, "Boy, do we have work to do here!"

When the class was over, I saw the scared look in people's eyes. It was a fear that derived not from what I'd told them or taught them, but from what they'd learned about how out of shape they were. When we returned the following week, ten people had dropped out; the week after that, we lost twelve more. When asked why they hadn't returned, people said they had "other things to do," a response that provided one of my primary motivations for wanting to educate people about the importance of learning personal protection techniques.

When I told this story recently during one of my Training for Life events, I was amazed to discover that one of my students from that course was in the room. She told me that she'd been one of the people who dropped out after the first week, and that the class had made her realize how truly vulnerable she really was. Her response was to figure that if she just kept a low profile and went about her business, she wouldn't be victimized. Unfortunately, however, that proved to be wrong.

She teared up a bit as she went on to say that, several years before, she'd met the person who she'd thought was going to be her soul mate but who turned out to be her worst nightmare instead. For her entire life, she said, she'd avoided even reading anything or watching any news broadcast that dealt with violence or victimization. She'd been living, as she put it, "in a bubble," and when she became involved with a man who physically assaulted and mentally abused her over a period of years, her bubble burst. She told me that the one thing she'd retained from her one day in my course was my having said that "the body has a self-preservation alarm, and when it goes off you have to answer it if you don't want to fall prey to the abuse you're encountering." Finally, she said, she answered the alarm. She had the man arrested, took out a restraining order against him, and eventually saw that he went to prison. Now she had come to the Training for Life event in order to finish what she'd started. Afterwards, we spoke privately, and she enrolled in one of my personal protection courses for women involved in domestic violence.

Fitness and Self-Defense Training

One of the questions I'm asked most frequently is how fit a person has to be in order to enroll in a martial-arts or self-defense course.

Mastering a martial art, as I've already said, requires not only focus and physical endurance but also a commitment of time. Other types of self-defense classes often include a variety of fitness drills to build up the body in order to endure in a fight.

Being in shape is always good, but self-defense instructors need to realize that training a person to deal with a random attack is very different from training someone to go head-to-head in a fight or a competition. I believe that a seasoned street fighter or seasoned Bad Guy will almost always prevail in a fight with a non-seasoned adversary. Properly trained, however, a non-seasoned adversary, a good everyday person, will be able to escape an attack and get to safety without being in tip-top shape.

Once self-defense instructors learn to stop saying, "You need to get in shape or you will never be able to defend yourself," society will, I believe, be more likely to embrace personal protection classes as a part of their daily lifestyle. An easy drill such as squeezing a soft rubber ball several hundred times a day will not only condition your hand but also release stress as you're doing it. Standing against a wall and getting up on your toes and then down at least fifty times a day will build up your calves. Holding on to a chair and lowering yourself to the ground by bending your knees will build up your legs. Little exercises like this will help train your hands to grab and your legs to get you away from an assailant, which is what the CDT system is all about.

I polled more than 1,000 martial-arts schools around the United States, and found that at each school, at any given time, there are on average fewer than fifteen students enrolled in any self-defense, or what I term self-protection, classes these schools offer. Many people seem to think that self-protection classes are some kind of watered-down version of the martial arts, but that simply isn't true. Any martial art, to be done correctly, takes years and years to master. Self-defense techniques may be borrowed from a specific martial art or from a combination of arts, and are taught in a basic short form that the average person can learn and retain and put into use under pressure. Many of these techniques do involve attacking the vitals, but most of the victims I've interviewed during the course of my career have indicated that, even though they did have some kind of training, they didn't fight back.

One such story was recounted by a female flight attendant for a major airline, who attended a Training for Life event I gave in Sacramento. The incident occurred when she'd completed a long day of flying and had checked into the hotel where she was staying overnight. She decided to visit a friend who lived nearby, and asked the concierge at her hotel if the address was within walking distance. He told her it was less than a half-mile from the hotel, and wrote out directions. She then called her friend to say she'd be there in half an hour, and she set out. It was a beautiful late-summer evening, and she'd just completed a three-hour self-defense course sanctioned by her airline, so she felt confident in her ability to take care of herself and was looking forward to the walk. On the way she stopped in a coffee shop to pick up a cup of coffee to go. When she came out and turned the corner, she was confronted by a man who said, "Hey, little lady, how about some company?" "No!" she said emphatically, and kept on walking. He then grabbed her arm and

IF YOUR MIND IS TRAINED, YOUR BODY WILL FOLLOW

The CDT system is designed for the average, everyday person and is based on using a minimal output of energy to achieve maximum results. I don't teach people how to win fights; I teach them how to escape from altercations. Whatever their shape, size, or degree of fitness, my students learn how to use their mental capacity to energize their physical capacity so that their minds and bodies are able to work together as a cohesive unit.

TOM'S TIP

said, "Don't be rude to a guy like me, because I hold your life in my hands."

At that point her survival instinct kicked in. She'd been taught in her class to take out the eyes, hit the throat, attack the groin, then finish the job. When she looked into this man's eyes, however, she said, "They looked so beady and small and sunken into his head that there was no way I could get to them." She then looked at his throat and saw that it was not exposed, as it had been when she learned the technique in class. He was also wearing baggy pants, and she felt that if she went for his groin and missed, he would surely kill her. Suddenly the confidence she'd gained from taking that self-defense class evaporated into thin air.

The guy then stated that he "owned the block," and walking on it would cost her her purse and all its contents. She gave him the purse and begged him not to hurt her. He then made her throw her shoes down a sewer grate and sit in the bushes until he was out of sight. She must have sat there crying for twenty minutes, she said, before she could gather the courage to get up and find a phone to call her friend. Together they went to the police station and filed a report, and her friend then took her back to the hotel.

When she met with her flight crew the next morning and told them what had happened, they asked if she'd thought of using her newly acquired self-defense techniques. Her reply was simple: "They taught us what to do and how to do it, but they didn't teach us that the criminal is scary, mean, and uses intimidation to create fear."

She then asked me if I thought she'd done the right thing. I told her what I tell all my clients: "Never defend a material possession, no matter how valuable you think it is or what it means to you. Defend yourself only when your life depends on it."

When she asked whether I thought she'd been trained properly, I said that what she'd been trained for was an encounter with a potential terrorist or an irate passenger on her airline, and that those situations were very different from encountering a Bad Guy on the street. It would be easier to turn a street criminal into a good person than to turn a good person into a Bad Guy. She told me that her class had been based on Special Forces training, and that she'd been taught to fight back rather than defend herself and escape. I teach the philosophy "less is better." I believe in giving people just enough awareness and skill to defend themselves and escape an altercation or potentially life-threatening situation. So my advice would be that if you're looking for a self-defense course, make sure it's based on escaping your attacker rather than annihilating him.

SELF-DEFENSE DEVICES AND HOW THEY WORK—OR DON'T WORK

The more conscious people become of the need for self-protection, the more they want to be educated about what types of devices are available to them, how they work, and, far from least important, if they are legal. Here's a list of some of the more popular devices and why I think they will—or will not—help you in a potentially life-threatening situation.

Personal Sound Alarm This is a box about the size of a hand, which looks more or less like a radio. It has a small strap that connects to a pin, and when you pull the strap the pin releases and emits a very loud and piercing sound. In one of my seminars, I asked five women who said they had these devices if they'd ever used them. Three of the women said they'd never used theirs and most of the time they just left them in the car because they were such a nuisance to carry. When I asked how often they changed the batteries, two of the three said they didn't even know the device worked off a battery, and the third said she'd had hers for three years and had never even checked to see if the battery was still working.

Of the two who had used the alarm, one said she'd thought she was being followed in her car and had set it off in the parking lot of a busy mall. Everyone stopped and looked around for a few seconds, but no one came to help her. The other woman said she'd used hers when two teenagers confronted her in the driveway of her home. One of them grabbed the alarm from her and smashed it against a wall. Then they robbed her and pushed her to the ground.

The problem, as I see it, is that the alarm itself isn't enough. You need to have a plan in place for what you're going to do after you set it off. Think about it. How often have you been walking on the street or in a parking lot and heard a car alarm go off? Did you hurry over to see if something was wrong? Did you use your cell phone to call 911? We've become accustomed to ignoring many sounds, and the sound of a car alarm is one of them. If you set off the alarm and then begin to scream and run yelling for help, I think—or hope—that someone will see you and help you. If you just set it off while you're being robbed or abducted, however, expect the criminal to grab it and smash it. An inexperienced criminal might get scared and run, but should he have a weapon and be chemically imbalanced, he might just pull the trigger. As in any unexpected or dangerous situation, you need to think before you act.

Pepper Spray This is a compound that gets into the eyes and face and burns the pores and membranes. The theory is that if you blind the Bad Guy, he won't be able to hurt you because he won't be able to see you. That's a good theory, but should it be taken away from you, or should the Bad Guy be carrying it himself, it could be used against you. It is, however, a weapon that's very popular among people who attend my seminars. But when I asked a thousand-member audience, only one person said she had used it, and that was to protect herself from a neighbor's dog.

When I asked how many had been robbed while carrying pepper spray, many people said they had. Why hadn't they used it, then? Well, some people said it was in their purse, and the Bad Guy had taken the purse. Others said they were afraid that if the Bad Guy took it away from them, he'd use it against them.

I asked the women in the audience if any of them had been assaulted by someone they knew or had feelings for, and three out of every five said they had. When I asked if they'd had pepper spray in the house, many said no, they kept it in the car. Among those who did have it in the house, many said it was in their purse or attached to their key chain and they were so frightened during the assault that they'd forgotten all about it.

Not one of the women knew the shelf life of the product or whether the spray they had was still good.

Personally, I think pepper spray can be useful if you've been trained in how to use it. The canisters come in all shapes and sizes, and can be hidden in various parts of the house just in case you encounter an intruder or if someone you know turns into a Bad Guest. You should also know that some types of spray will work from up to six feet away, so it can be a good distance weapon. Always remember to keep these sprays somewhere that children can't get to them, and know what to do if you or one of your family members accidentally gets sprayed with it.

Pulse Waves These are handheld devices that were developed from the new science of pulse-wave technology. To use the pulse wave, you have to press a button and push the device against the assailant's body, so that it intercepts his brain waves and scrambles the nervous system. As I understand it, the assailant will then become immobilized and collapse to the ground so that you can get away.

HOW TO BUY AND USE PEPPER SPRAY

- Purchase a can that fits comfortably in your hand.

- Choose one that's small enough to be concealed in your hand.

- Make a fist around the canister, with the spray end pointed away from you. If the release button is on the top, press it with your thumb; if it's on the side, like the trigger of a gun, press the trigger with your index finger.

- Always spray low to high so that, if he tries to duck, your attacker will walk directly into it. If you spray too high, it might go right over his head, allowing him to rush you and grab the spray.

- Never carry pepper spray or keep it in your home unless you know how to use it properly.

TOM'S TIP

I have to say that I've never had any personal experience with this particular device, but to me it sounds like a modern version of a stun gun. And since it requires that you get in close and make physical contact with your assailant, you must be able to use it properly and without hesitation or fear in a pressured situation. Should it be taken away from you, it would make the Bad Guy's job a lot easier.

Blow-Up People During a seminar I held recently in Texas, I was asked about the efficacy of using blow-up people—inflatable mannequins—in your car. My answer is that if you're a private detective on a stakeout and you dress the doll up to make it look more like a person, it might help. But I think that most of these dolls are highly unrealistic and wouldn't do much to fool a potential assailant. The woman who asked the question at my seminar said they were intended to prevent abductions while driving. Since most carjacking victims are driving alone, I suppose it might be a deterrent, but if the potential carjacker actually opened the door or got a close look, he'd immediately see that your companion was made out of rubber. Frankly, I think these blow-up people are really rather silly and can be a waste of money.

Keys Many self-defense courses are now teaching people how common, everyday objects such as keys, rings, and pens can be used as weapons to take out an attacker's eyes or stab him in the throat. At a Training for Life event in Texas, one woman who had taken such a course told me a story about what had happened to her the previous winter when she was leaving her company's holiday party. On her way through the parking lot, she decided to take out her keys and insert one between each of her fingers, as she'd been taught in class, so that if she were attacked she could jab her way to freedom. As she was scanning her surroundings for anyone who might be lurking in the shadows, she slipped and fell on a patch of black ice. Automatically, she braced herself to avoid hitting her face, and, in doing that, she fell directly on the keys, stabbing herself underneath her chin and cutting her hand in several places.

Luckily, one of her co-workers was there to call an ambulance. "We were taught that keys could do damage," she said, "but what we weren't taught was to watch not only our surroundings but also where and how we were walking." Now, although she believes the keys might help her in defense of her life, she doesn't carry them because of the memory she has of what it felt like when the keys drove into her chin. "I don't think I could purposely do that to another human being," she told me.

Blinding Light Like the pulse wave, this is a modern weapon based on putting so much candlepower into a flashlight-type device that shining it into the eyes of an attacker will blind him for several minutes. I've watched a video demonstrating how the device can be used in various law-enforcement situations. It seemed like a useful tool, but I do have some questions about it. For one thing, the de-

HOW TO HOLD KEYS DEFENSIVELY

Pick the longest key with the greatest number of jagged edges. Lodge it, pointing outward, in the V between your thumb and your index finger, with the rest of your keys clutched in your palm. Squeeze your hand into a fist to hold it securely. The key now becomes a jabbing tool to use with a natural motion, like inserting a key in a lock, and minimal risk of cutting your own hand.

TOM'S TIP

vice shown in the video was too large for the average person to carry comfortably on his or her person, and there was no indication that it was available in smaller models. For another, it was not made clear how close you would have to be to your assailant to make it effective, or whether other people in the area would also be blinded. And if a child inadvertently shone it into his own eyes, what might be the long-term effect? Finally, as with any of these devices, concealment and access to the light at the moment you need it are the keys to its efficacy.

Stun Guns I was at a training seminar for law-enforcement personnel when I decided to volunteer to find out what getting zapped by a stun gun would feel like. It was literally a shocking experience, to say the least, and I do believe that in the right—well-trained—hands, stun guns can be extremely effective weapons. People whom I've asked said they'd never purchased one because they weren't sure they'd have the nerve to use it and they were afraid the Bad Guy or Bad Guest would take it away and use it against them.

My two biggest concerns about stun guns are, first, that a child might accidentally get hold of one, and, second, that they're illegal in many states.

Several criminals I interviewed said they had actually stolen a purse that turned out to contain a stun gun. When that happened, they sold the device to a teenage gang member on the street who undoubtedly then used it to rob someone else!

Bladed Weapons Many people ask whether I think it's a good idea for them to carry an edged weapon such as a knife or a box cutter. My answer is that if you're trained to use it, a bladed weapon can be an extremely useful self-defense tool, but if you're not, it can be a deadly mistake. You have to realize that, in order to use a knife, you have to be very close to the person against whom you're using it. Sticking something sharp into another human being is difficult enough for trained military personnel, much less the average citizen. And, unlike other weapons, a knife must enter the right place at the right angle in order to stop a person in his tracks. I would say that if it's a matter of life or death, using a knife might be a choice of last resort, but before you decide to keep one in your vehicle or on your person, you'd be wise to give the matter a great deal of thought.

The following story was told to me by a seasoned criminal who had spent most of his life in and out of prison. One day during the holiday season he decided to randomly target a female victim in the parking lot of a shopping center and rob her of her purchases, her jewelry, and her purse.

He waited at the rear of the shopping center, where there were no lights and the concrete walls would block the sound of crying or screaming. The vehicle he chose to wait by was at the very back of the lot, near the railroad tracks, which were hidden behind a line of pine trees that would also provide good cover. Soon a woman came out carrying shopping bags and singing "Holly Jolly Christmas." As she approached the car, he pinned her against the door, as if they were just having a conversation. He told her he had a gun in his pocket and demanded that she drop her shopping bags next to her feet, and then remove her jewelry and put it in one of the bags along with her purse.

The woman spoke calmly, saying that she just wanted her driver's license and her Social Security card, and that he was welcome to everything else. She then reached into her purse, but instead of removing her identification, she pulled out a knife, backed up, and said, "If you come near me, I will cut you."

Instead of running, however, the robber got mad—very mad. After making a few rude comments, he moved in and punched her in the face, knocking her to the ground and the knife out of her hand. He then grabbed both the knife and the hand in which she'd held it, and cut her hand several times. As a parting shot, he said, "If you pull a knife, you'd better be prepared to use it, especially against a guy like me." Then he spit on her, grabbed her valuables, and walked nonchalantly away. He was eventually caught and spent several years in prison for the crime. The woman, according to the assailant, received fifty stitches in her hand.

Firearms Owning a firearm for so-called home protection is one thing; carrying one on your person is quite another. In either case, a gun, unlike a knife, can be used from a distance. You pull the trigger, the bullet leaves the barrel, and that's that. But, unless you're highly trained, you won't have much control over where that bullet is going, and you just might hit an innocent bystander or a loved one.

It's very difficult in many states to obtain a permit to carry a handgun for self-protection, and doing so without a permit might just get you a mandatory jail term. In addition, if a police officer sees you carrying a gun, he might think you are a criminal. If you're nervous and, in your anxiety to prove your innocence, you appear to be reaching for your weapon, he might just shoot you in what he considers self-defense. And in such an instance, he would be justified.

Using a gun also requires that you have access to it. Walking the streets carrying it in your hand is obviously not an option. It's a fact that when a home is robbed, one of the items most often stolen is a firearm. The robber then either uses it for his own purposes or sells it on the street for extra cash. Keeping a weapon in your car, in your purse, or by your bed might make it more easily accessible to you in certain instances, but it might make it more accessible to the Bad Guy as well.

SELF-DEFENSE SAFETY

- Whatever self-defense tool you are carrying, keep it out of sight, either cupped in your hand, if it's small enough, or in your coat pocket.
- Use it only if your life depends on it. No material possession is worth the risk of your life or that of a loved one.
- Think before you act and, when acting, use the safest defense possible with the quickest, most natural motion.
- Don't carry anything you are afraid to use. It will only come back to haunt you should you meet a Bad Guy who turns abusive and uses your self-defense weapon against you.

TOM'S TIP

And, of course, there's the issue of children gaining access to firearms and causing tragic accidents. The child is not to blame for playing with the weapon; it's the parents or guardians who are at fault for not giving the weapon the respect it deserves, and for leaving it in a place where the child can get to it.

CDT—COMPLIANCE, DIRECTION, TAKEDOWN

If the martial arts are too time-consuming and strenuous, and don't give people the confidence they need to use them outside a controlled environment; if military-type self-defense courses teach skills too violent and combative for the average person to comprehend, much less put into practice; and if self-defense devices are often inaccessible or as likely to backfire as to save us in an altercation, then what is the good guy trying to navigate safely through a world of Bad Guys, Bad Guests, and Bad Situations to do?

My answer was to seek a less violent approach. The result has been the development of my personal philosophy of defense, Train-

TEMPORARY EFFECTS OF CDT TECHNIQUES

- temporary pain to a targeted area
- temporary immobilization of targeted area
- momentary loss of equilibrium
- momentary malfunction of direct motor skills
- temporary mental dysfunction
- possible muscle cramping

ing for Life, which is based on a Stun and Run technique. My system uses simple movements with which we are all familiar, and is based on short-circuiting the non-vital, superficial nerve systems that are closest to the skin. It takes no more than the weight of a dime to block the direct path of a nerve, and by taking that pressure one step further, using a pinch, grab, pull, twist, or insert, it is possible to shut down the impulse nerve temporarily, thereby interrupting an attacker's motion and providing an opportunity for the intended victim to escape. What I teach my students is "confuse, then leave." In other words, confuse your attacker by short-circuiting the signals the nervous system sends to the brain, and then get away as quickly and noisily as you can. Less is better. The less force you need to expend, the less wear and tear on your body, the less mental stress, and the less time it takes to escape unharmed, the better the system is working.

In developing my system, I focused on eight points that would have to be met in order for me to consider it a success:

1. It would not be barbaric and would be based on nonlethal force, which would be more appealing—and easier—for most people to learn. It would take into account the reasons the average person doesn't train in the martial arts or self-defense, and thus would not be a martial art.

2. It would have to be based on everyday movements we already know, so that the techniques would be easy to learn and easy to remember.

3. It would be based on an escape mentality, teaching how to get out of harm's way as quickly and safely as possible.

4. The techniques would have to work for the majority of people, regardless of gender, size, or physical conditioning.

5. The techniques would have to work together in various combinations depending upon the situation as well as each individual's ability and comfort level.

6. It would be as effortless as possible, using a "less is better" philosophy.

7. It would have to be based on the lawful use of force, so that no one would wind up in prison or lose his or her assets as the result of a lawsuit. Most attacks are nonlethal and don't call for the escalation of force that is being taught in so many self-defense classes today.

8. It would have to have a name everyone could remember, because when the mind retains something, so does the body.

CDT—Compliance (controlling, countering, or defusing the attack or attacker), Direction (directing the attack or attacker out of the way in order to escape), Takedown (taking the attacker to the ground to give you more time to escape, or holding him there if no other option is available)—meets all of those criteria. It's a proven system that can work for everyone. The movements don't require power or special skills. They are all based on grabbing, squeezing, pulling, and turning—movements we all use every day when we're turning a key, knocking on a door, or wringing out a washcloth.

While most systems of self-defense are based on a "stay and annihilate" philosophy that, for anyone who is not extremely well trained, can turn into the nightmare of nightmares, mine is based on a "stun and run" system that uses the body's natural instinct to flee when cornered or harmed.

In my classes I ask people to run or walk quickly from one end of the training center to the other while I time them. Then I simu-

FEAR IS YOUR FRIEND AND PRESSURE IS YOUR ALLY

Studies have proved that fear is a stronger emotion than love. That said, however, we tend to avoid rather than embrace our fears. CDT training allows you to face your fear in a controlled situation and use it for motivation while, at the same time, you learn the technique for applying just the right type and amount of pressure—meaning physical pressure on a targeted area of an assailant's body, as you're about to see—required for self-defense.

TOM'S TIP

late a surprise attack on the same people and again time their movement over the same distance. In most cases they move twice as fast after being attacked than they did in a nonstressful situation.

My philosophy is that he or she who runs today will live to run another day. Based on my research and experience, I have come up with what I call "the twenty-foot barrier," which means that once a victim has run twenty feet while screaming or otherwise drawing attention to himself, the Bad Guy or Bad Guest will usually flee to avoid being caught.

Because your mind and body are working together for your protection, it's important that you approach self-defense with the proper mindset. You must be mentally prepared to defend yourself, and the best attitude to take is one of resentment. Send your attacker mental messages such as "You have to be nuts to put your hands on me!" or "There is no way you're going to dictate the course of my life!" You're in defense mode now, and you need to remember that if you can't, he can! If you can't defend yourself, he can do whatever he wants and you will no longer control your own destiny. Your motivation is to retain control of your life.

Listed below are five basic CDT techniques I teach in my Training for Life courses. They are based on disrupting the statistically most common forms of attack the average person will encounter.

THE HANDS DO THE MOTION; THE MIND GIVES YOU THE PROCESS

Many victims have told me that they felt a surge of energy when they were attacked, but wasted it because they didn't know what to do. Your hands *want* to defend your body, and CDT trains your mind to send the proper signals so that the energy of your hands won't be wasted.

TOM'S TIP

THE V-TRIGGER

This technique is most useful if a Bad Guest (or a Bad Guy) should grab you by the arm, wrist, or hand. It isn't any more difficult to learn than rapping sharply on a door with your knuckle. The key to making the technique work is to keep your fist tightly closed in a knocking position and make sure that when you apply your force you do it hard, because your life depends on it. Imagine that you are knocking on the door to a house where there is loud music playing inside. You have to knock hard and loud in order to be heard—just as the force of your "knock" has to penetrate deeply enough to cause your assailant to let you go.

WHEN TO USE IT When an assailant grabs you by the arm, wrist, or hand, and your other hand is free. It is also good to have a backup to your technique. In this case the Shin Insertion (page 226) is a perfect match.

EVERYDAY MOTION TO REMEMBER Knocking on a door.

WHY IT WORKS You are changing the impulse in a nerve located in the middle of the front part of the hand, which will cause the attacker to open his hand reflexively and release his grip.

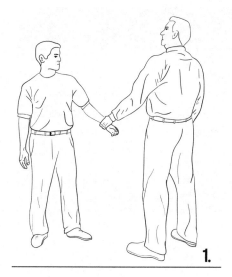

1.

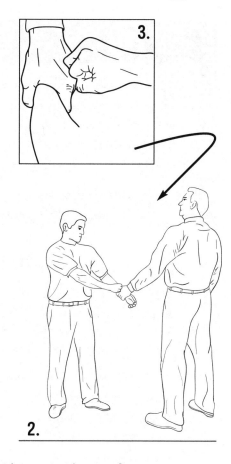

3.

2.

HOW TO DO IT

1. Make a fist with your thumb either inside or outside your fingers. Make sure it is very tight.

2. Look for the spot on the back of your attacker's hand that is directly below the V formed by the first and second fingers and close to the knuckles. Any part of the hand will work, but the area closest to the second and third knuckles is the most sensitive.

3. Rap the point sharply with your knuckle. Don't be shy—you want that door to open, so knock hard. Your attacker will immediately let go.

4. Turn around, YELL to draw attention to yourself, and run to increase the distance between you and your attacker! The more distance you can create, the less likely it is that he'll attack again.

LET HIM COMMIT

Since most attacks are up close and personal, the Bad Guy or Bad Guest will want to intimidate you by grabbing you. Understand your skill and your objective. Let him commit. Once his hands are tied up, yours will be free to do the job of protecting you. That's when you need to see the window of opportunity, apply the pressure, and get out the door.

TOM'S TIP

UPPER-ARM INSERTION

WHEN TO USE IT If you are grabbed by your lapel, hair, or throat, and at least one hand is free. Again, use the Shin Insertion (page 226) as your backup. Since the focus of the assailant will be on your upper body, it is very unlikely that he will see the Shin Insertion coming.

EVERYDAY MOTION TO REMEMBER Turning a key.

WHY IT WORKS You're disrupting the superficial nerves located in the fleshy skin between the muscle groups on the upper arm, which will cause your attacker to release his grip.

HOW TO DO IT

1. Feel along the inside of the attacker's upper arm until you reach the soft skin. The closer you get to the armpit, the better this will work.

2. Grab the skin and pull down so the skin is tight. Keeping the skin tight and compressed, turn your hand as hard as you can in either a clockwise or counterclockwise direction as you pull downward at a 45-degree angle. His grasp will immediately release. Do not let go until he releases you. Remember, you are grabbing the superficial layer of skin, so the less you grab, the better the technique.

3. Now run and create distance, and don't forget to yell and draw attention to yourself and the situation.

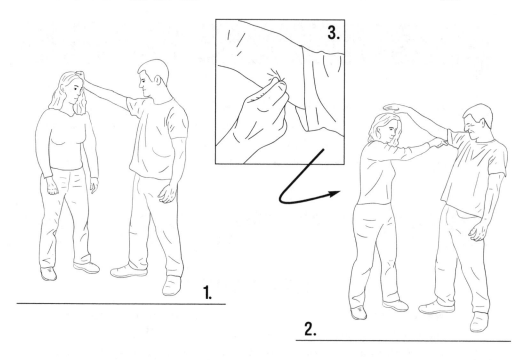

INSERT, DON'T PUNCH

Punching is not a natural motion, but poking and prodding motions, which I call insertions, are. That's why they are so easy to learn and so effective.

I've interviewed many victims who were never taught how to punch, or, if they were, never practiced what they'd been taught. As a result, when they got into an altercation and threw a punch, it either missed the target or they broke their hand, which left them defenseless and pleading for mercy.

Our hands and fingers are very agile and, when properly trained, can be extremely effective defense weapons. Remember, the hand is quicker than the eye; all CDT training does is show you how to use it correctly.

TOM'S TIP

WHEN TO HOLD YOUR BREATH

If someone grabs you by the throat, don't panic because you think you can't breathe. Instead hold your breath as you naturally would when swimming. In fact, you naturally hold your breath all the time, in various situations, usually without even being aware of it. The average person can hold her breath well over thirty seconds, which is much longer than the time you'll need to initiate your release.

TOM'S TIP

SHIN INSERTION

WHEN TO USE IT If you've been grabbed from the front (it also can be modified to use when you're grabbed from behind, but for now let's concentrate on the front because statistically that is the most likely scenario), by the shoulders, throat, hair, or clothing; if your hands are not free; or if your attacker is wearing a heavy coat or you can't get a good enough grip to apply the Upper-Arm Insertion. If your assailant doesn't let you go, do it again with the opposite leg and don't stop doing it until you are freed.

EVERYDAY MOTION TO REMEMBER Think of a low-level kick, the kind you would use playing kickball or soccer. The movement is that of lifting your toe and dragging your heel, which is something many people do every day. If you look at the bottom of your shoe, you'll probably see that the back of the heel is worn down, which means that you naturally drag your heels when you walk.

WHY IT WORKS The shinbone is very close to the skin, giving easy access to the sensitive nerve centers. Temporarily disrupting those nerves will start a chain reaction that causes the attacker to release his grip.

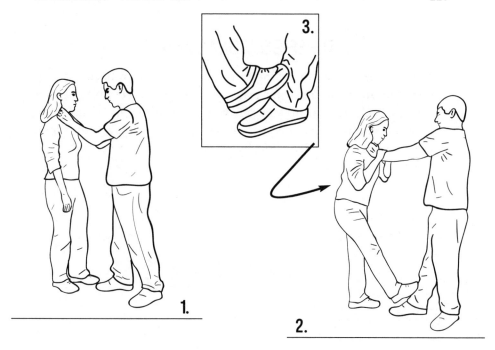

HOW TO DO IT

1. Drag your foot up in a natural motion at a 45-degree angle to get your toe up and into the shin. Do this as if you were walking, but instead of picking your foot up and placing it down, drag it upward from the toe to the heel.

2. Generate as much force as you can, aimed directly into the shin. Because the shin is one of the most sensitive parts of the body, this will disrupt your attacker's nervous system, causing him to let go.

3. Now run, scream, or yell to draw attention to yourself and try to get as far away from the attacker as possible!

THREE-SECTIONAL ANGLE

WHEN TO USE IT You can use this technique if you are grabbed in a bear hug from the front and your arms are free. If you are able, step far enough back from your attacker, you can use this in combination with the Shin Insertion. Or, if your attacker is holding you too close, use a modified Shin Insertion by scraping your foot up and down against his shinbone.

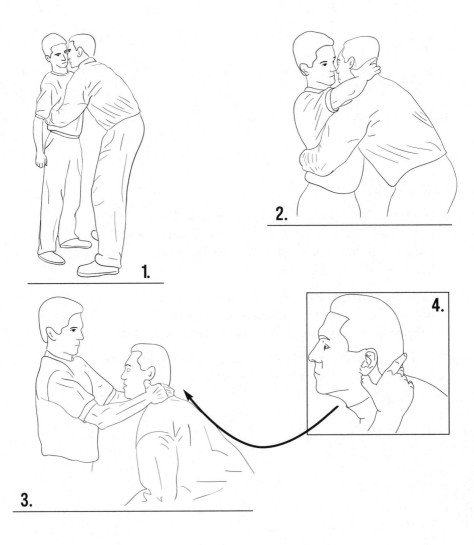

EVERYDAY MOTION TO REMEMBER The best way to see this motion is to think of clasping your hands together so that, when your palms meet, your thumbs bend and cross and your fingers naturally lock. The position of your thumbs would be the same as when you're kneading dough or pushing the buttons on your TV's remote control with one hand.

WHY IT WORKS The nerves behind the ears are extremely sensitive. Disrupting the signals from those nerves interrupts the attacker's thought process, creating a temporary loss of equilibrium, which will cause him to release his grip.

HOW TO DO IT

1. Locate the three-sectional angle, which is the cavity or gap located directly behind the lower ear, parallel to where the earlobe begins.

2. Bend your fingers slightly, which will keep your hands strong and generate more power for prodding.

3. Insert your thumbs or middle fingers into the cavities or gaps behind your attacker's ears, the three-sectional angle.

4. Drive your fingers in as hard as you can at a 45-degree angle, pushing one thumb up and the other down in order to disrupt and confuse your attacker's nervous system, causing him to let go.

5. Turn around, run, yell, draw attention to yourself, and get out of there.

LOWER INSERTION POINT

This is the point on the inner thigh, similar to the point on the inner arm, where there is soft skin between two muscle groups.

WHEN TO USE IT When your attacker is on top of you, straddling you, choking you, or hitting you. If your hands are free and you can reach your assailant's head, you can do this in combination with the Three-Sectional Angle.

EVERYDAY MOTION TO REMEMBER This motion is the same as turning a key, but requires grabbing more area and uses greater strength, so think about opening a jar that is stuck.

WHY IT WORKS This technique is very effective because it grabs many nerves at once. Turning hard and fast then creates a temporary traffic jam to all those nerve centers, causing the assailant to lose his equilibrium so that you are able to use the weight of his body as leverage to rotate or push him off you.

HOW TO DO IT

1. Run your fingers up the inner thigh until you feel soft skin. The higher you go, the more sensitive the nervous system and the more effective the technique.

2. Grab with your entire hand and twist as hard as you can, as if you were opening a stubborn jar or turning a key with added force. As you do this, use the weight of your attacker's now-destabilized body as leverage to rotate him off you.

3. Should the situation dictate, you can hold the attacker in this position as long as you need to simply by maintaining your grip, but your first choice should always be to escape as quickly as possible.

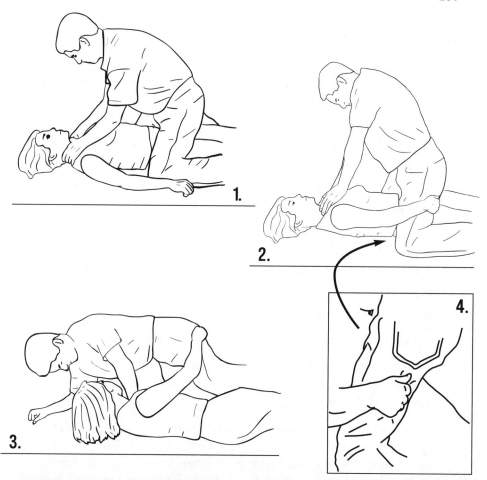

A LITTLE ACTING GOES A LONG WAY

Letting your attacker believe you're in pain and afraid, even a little pleading while you're planning the best technique to use for the particular situation you're in, can cause him to let down his guard and make your job a bit easier. Other than that, however, you should *never* talk to your attacker. Talking will slow down your reactions by at least one-eighth of a second, which could mean the difference between grabbing and losing your all-important window of opportunity.

TOM'S TIP

CHECKLIST FOR USING CDT TECHNIQUES

✔ When you're in a serious situation, you need to get serious. Don't be tentative. Apply these techniques with the intent and understanding that your life depends on them.

✔ Always deal with the moment. Don't allow yourself to feel self-pity or self-doubt. Believe in your training and never stop until you are out of harm's way.

✔ Unless you're highly trained, don't punch or kick; insert, grab, and squeeze.

✔ Use any combination of these techniques that works for you. Mix and match if you can. CDT techniques are based on the same principles as a good marriage, which means they all work well with one another.

✔ Defuse the situation as quickly as possible, then leave.

✔ Get away. Don't stop to look at what you've done. Just get away!

✔ Remember to scream, yell, and draw attention to yourself. The more people who see you and hear you, the better your chances that someone will help you.

✔ Practice makes perfect, and if you're practicing a technique that may one day save your life, it's certainly worth the time. You can practice in your mind by visualizing the techniques whenever you have a free minute. Picture yourself doing it successfully and getting away safely. You can also practice physically with another adult whom you trust. Just remember that you are doing this to help, not hurt one another.

Very Important Never attempt to perform these techniques with children unless or until you have completed an actual CDT or Training for Life course. Their nervous systems are not fully developed and you may be too strong for their smaller body mass to withstand. Once you have successfully completed a CDT or Training for Life course and have a thorough understanding of how the techniques work, you will be better able to practice with your children.

STAYING SAFE: IT'S IN YOUR HANDS

ABOUT TEN YEARS AGO *I had a student named Mike who, after taking a few classes, decided to get his fiancée, Valerie, involved as well so that they'd have something they could do together. Both Mike and Valerie were wonderful, enthusiastic, attractive people. No matter what else might have been going on in her life, Valerie always got to class on time, and no matter how hard I pushed her, she gave it her all and kept on smiling.*

One day Mike couldn't come to class and Valerie brought a girlfriend along instead. It happened that they were the only two students there that day, so we concentrated on personal defense for women. Valerie and her friend had a wonderful time beating me up, but, even though they were laughing, they paid attention to what I was teaching.

After class I took them both for pizza, and as we were happily munching away, Valerie told me about her plans for the future. She would marry Mike and have a family. She wanted lots of kids and lots of dogs, and her goal was to be the ideal mother. After our conversation, I walked the women to their car, and Valerie hugged me good-bye, saying, "I always thought you were a tough guy, but you're really a good guy." I told her not to spread it around or she'd ruin my reputation, and then we parted ways.

The next night, while driving in a rainstorm, Valerie was involved in an accident and died instantly. My question was "Why?" And most of all, "Why her?"

○ ○ ○

AS I'VE COME TO LEARN both personally and professionally, life is both sacred and fragile, and we must do all we can to preserve it.

Bad Guys and Bad Guests are "bad" in the sense that they have chosen to act in ways that are not only against the law but also against our basic human instincts to be good, law-abiding citizens who are considerate of one another. That doesn't mean, however, that they are necessarily unintelligent. If they're good at what they do, it's often because they realize that the majority of us so-called solid citizens lack even the most basic awareness, safety, and personal protection skills, and, because of that, we effectively offer ourselves up to be victimized.

What we all need to realize is that while certain styles, enthusiasms, and interests may be here today and gone tomorrow, personal protection is not a fad; it is a skill we need to learn, develop, and practice throughout our lives. Our minds and bodies can learn most things we ask of them because they are both designed to live and function, and they have wonderful mechanisms for self-preservation. We, however, have a duty to teach our minds and bodies the techniques of personal protection just as we teach our children their ABCs or ourselves how to dance or swim.

If the majority of good people in this country and around the world made it their responsibility to become more safety-conscious, there would be more good, trained people looking out for one another, and we would all be safer as a result. There are, without doubt, more good people than bad in this world. What we need, however, is to shift the balance by making sure that more of those good people are *trained* than *untrained*, because, as we've so tragically learned, the Bad Guys will almost certainly be well trained. And isn't it better to know something and not need to use it than to need it and not know it, especially when your life or that of a loved one depends on that knowledge?

Think about it this way. Anywhere you go, most of the people around you, whatever their size, shape, color, or gender, are good people who, if they were armed with the right knowledge, could and would help someone in trouble. The real reason there aren't more good Samaritans around is that they just don't have the training. They may have good intentions, but they lack the skills to back them up. My mission is to spread the word that it's time to become a safer nation. Each one of the people at my CDT centers and all the people involved in the Tom Patire Training for Life campaign are and will be educated to be ABP—able-bodied people." The more ABP there are, the better chance we have to look out for each other. My mission, and that of the thousands of instructors who have joined the Training for Life cause, is to educate the public about how to be safe and being prepared.

When I was doing a show for Fox TV some time back, one of the people who interviewed me before my appearance asked how I would define my mission in life. I told her that I, along with my friend and mentor, Dave Geliebter, had taken on a task at which many people had failed. Simply put, it was to make people more aware—aware of their surroundings, of their responsibility for ensuring their own safety, of the options that were open to them for doing that, and of how to acquire the skills they would need.

More recently, we hired Mark Amuso of Dylan Durango Consulting to organize my national Training for Life campaign. Initially, Mark's reaction to what I was doing was to say, "Fear turns people off." As he watched, however, he learned soon enough that what I'm all about is not increasing people's fears, but banishing them by helping people to develop confidence in their skills and the positive mindset that will keep them and their loved ones safe in the smartest, most legal way ever developed. Training for Life has never been based on fear. Rather, it is based on spreading the word—and that word is *empowerment*. Safety lies in preparation, and depends on knowledge that can be turned into skill.

A television personality once nicknamed me "Guardian of Safety." At first I thought it was just a name, but I now realize that it's the right name for a man with a mission—a personal-protection mission—and I wear it proudly.

Be safe!

TOM PATIRE'S PLEDGE OF AWARENESS

I hereby do swear

To live my life being prepared,

To put safety first for everyone to see,

By caring for loved ones as well as for me.

To assure through my actions of not being scared

By making this Pledge: Always Be Aware!!

INDEX

For more information on Tom Patire's programs, or to order the Training for Life Video Series, call 1-888-237-7287 or visit www.tompatire.com or www.cdt-training.com.